Cumulative probabilities for the standard norma

z	0.00	0.01	0.02	0.03	0.04	0.05				
0.0	.5000	.5040	.5080	.5120	.5160	.5199				
0.1	.5398	.5438	.5478	.5517	.5557	.5596	[illegible]			
0.2	.5793	.5832	.5871	.5910	.5948	.5987	.6026	.6064	.6103	.6141
0.3	.6179	.6217	.6255	.6293	.6331	.6368	.6406	.6443	.6480	.6517
0.4	.6554	.6591	.6628	.6664	.6700	.6736	.6772	.6808	.6844	.6879
0.5	.6915	.6950	.6985	.7019	.7054	.7088	.7123	.7157	.7190	.7224
0.6	.7257	.7291	.7324	.7357	.7389	.7422	.7454	.7486	.7517	.7549
0.7	.7580	.7611	.7642	.7673	.7704	.7734	.7764	.7794	.7823	.7852
0.8	.7881	.7910	.7939	.7967	.7995	.8023	.8051	.8078	.8106	.8133
0.9	.8159	.8186	.8212	.8238	.8264	.8289	.8315	.8340	.8365	.8389
1.0	.8413	.8438	.8461	.8485	.8508	.8531	.8554	.8577	.8599	.8621
1.1	.8643	.8665	.8686	.8708	.8729	.8749	.8770	.8790	.8810	.8830
1.2	.8849	.8869	.8888	.8907	.8925	.8944	.8962	.8980	.8997	.9015
1.3	.9032	.9049	.9066	.9082	.9099	.9115	.9131	.9147	.9162	.9177
1.4	.9192	.9207	.9222	.9236	.9251	.9265	.9279	.9292	.9306	.9319
1.5	.9332	.9345	.9357	.9370	.9382	.9394	.9406	.9418	.9429	.9441
1.6	.9452	.9463	.9474	.9484	.9495	.9505	.9515	.9525	.9535	.9545
1.7	.9554	.9564	.9573	.9582	.9591	.9599	.9608	.9616	.9625	.9633
1.8	.9641	.9649	.9656	.9664	.9671	.9678	.9686	.9693	.9699	.9706
1.9	.9713	.9719	.9726	.9732	.9738	.9744	.9750	.9756	.9761	.9767
2.0	.9772	.9778	.9783	.9788	.9793	.9798	.9803	.9808	.9812	.9817
2.1	.9821	.9826	.9830	.9834	.9838	.9842	.9846	.9850	.9854	.9857
2.2	.9861	.9864	.9868	.9871	.9875	.9878	.9881	.9884	.9887	.9890
2.3	.9893	.9896	.9898	.9901	.9904	.9906	.9909	.9911	.9913	.9916
2.4	.9918	.9920	.9922	.9925	.9927	.9929	.9931	.9932	.9934	.9936
2.5	.9938	.9940	.9941	.9943	.9945	.9946	.9948	.9949	.9951	.9952
2.6	.9953	.9955	.9956	.9957	.9959	.9960	.9961	.9962	.9963	.9964
2.7	.9965	.9966	.9967	.9968	.9969	.9970	.9971	.9972	.9973	.9974
2.8	.9974	.9975	.9976	.9977	.9977	.9978	.9979	.9979	.9980	.9981
2.9	.9981	.9982	.9982	.9983	.9984	.9984	.9985	.9985	.9986	.9986
3.0	.9987	.9987	.9987	.9988	.9988	.9989	.9989	.9989	.9990	.9990
3.1	.9990	.9991	.9991	.9991	.9992	.9992	.9992	.9992	.9993	.9993
3.2	.9993	.9993	.9994	.9994	.9994	.9994	.9994	.9995	.9995	.9995
3.3	.9995	.9995	.9995	.9996	.9996	.9996	.9996	.9996	.9996	.9997
3.4	.9997	.9997	.9997	.9997	.9997	.9997	.9997	.9997	.9997	.9998
3.5	.9998	.9998	.9998	.9998	.9998	.9998	.9998	.9998	.9998	.9998
3.6	.9998	.9998	.9999	.9999	.9999	.9999	.9999	.9999	.9999	.9999
3.7	.9999	.9999	.9999	.9999	.9999	.9999	.9999	.9999	.9999	.9999
3.8	.9999	.9999	.9999	.9999	.9999	.9999	.9999	.9999	.9999	.9999

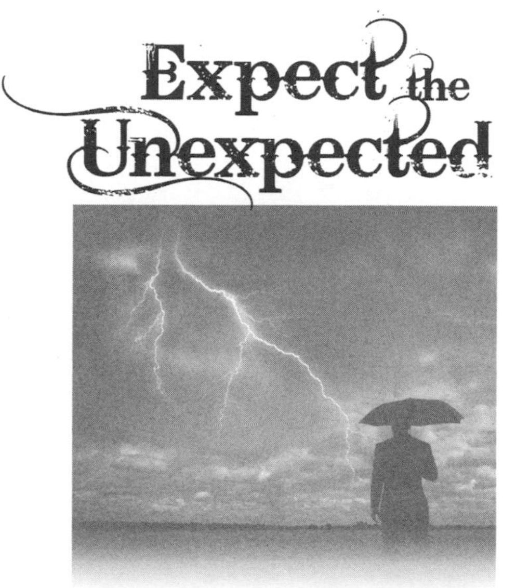

A First Course in Biostatistics

Expect the Unexpected

A First Course in Biostatistics

Raluca Balan • Gilles Lamothe

University of Ottawa, Canada

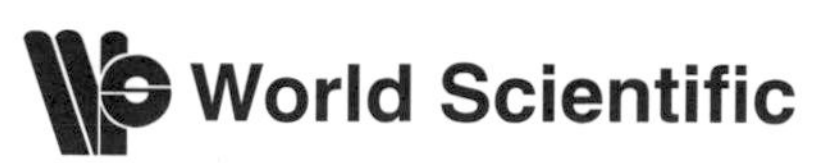

NEW JERSEY • LONDON • SINGAPORE • BEIJING • SHANGHAI • HONG KONG • TAIPEI • CHENNAI

Published by

World Scientific Publishing Co. Pte. Ltd.

5 Toh Tuck Link, Singapore 596224

USA office: 27 Warren Street, Suite 401-402, Hackensack, NJ 07601

UK office: 57 Shelton Street, Covent Garden, London WC2H 9HE

Library of Congress Cataloging-in-Publication Data

Balan, Raluca.

Expect the unexpected : a first course in biostatistics / Raluca Balan, Gilles Lamothe.

p. cm.

Includes bibliographical references.

ISBN-13 978-981-4291-32-3

ISBN-10 981-4291-32-3

1. Biometry -- Textbooks. 2. Probabilities. 3. Statistics. I. Title. II. Lamothe, Gilles.

QH323.5 .B353 2011

2011283713

British Library Cataloguing-in-Publication Data

A catalogue record for this book is available from the British Library.

First published 2011

Reprinted 2012

Printed in Singapore by World Scientific Printers.

Preface

Scholars have tried for many years to find the meaning of Hamlet's last words *"The Rest is Silence?"* in Shakespeare's play. In a 2007 movie with the same title as Hamlet's famous quote, in the city of Bucharest of 1911, a 19-year old actor decides to become a film director (an utopian dream at the time), after realizing that cinema could save for eternity some of the magic captured in a theater performance. The present book has been born from the desire to give an answer to the very same question, that we face at the end of each term when we finish teaching a course. Could it be possible to save for the future generations of students some parts of the vibrant atmosphere in the classroom and make them share this incredible experience?

This manuscript has been developed from the authors' lecture notes for the course MAT 2379 "Introduction to Biostatistics" (and its former counterpart MAT 2378 "Probability and Statistics for the Natural Sciences"), that has been taught at University of Ottawa since 2003 to the present. During the years, these notes have constantly evolved and been enriched with more examples; this process will probably continue over the years to come. However, most of the examples that are included in the book are new and have not been used in the classroom before.

Unless a source of information is specified, all the examples in the book are using hypothetical data. The examples are usually based on a real-life situation, which is connected in a very simple way to the natural sciences. Computer-generated data sets have been avoided, and simulation results are not discussed.

The goal of the book is to introduce and explore the usefulness of various statistical or probabilistic methods, by means of simple and non-technical examples, allowing the reader to understand quickly the meaning of a newly introduced concept, and apply it later in a more complex situation. Some of the examples used in the book are drawing the attention to various problems of today's world, related to environmental issues, climate change, loss of biodiversity, and their impact on wildlife and humans.

The book has two parts. Part I introduces the basic concepts and rules of probability theory, while Part II focuses on statistics. This order reflects the authors' philosophy that probability theory lies at the foundation of statistics, and that it is important to understand the meaning of randomness before doing any data analysis. This explains why the topic of descriptive statistics is discussed only in Part II, and not at the beginning, as it seems to be the common practice when teaching statistics.

In a 1914 address by Raymond Pearl to the American Statistical Society entitled "The Service and Importance of Statistics to Biology", he mentioned three important contributions of statistical methods to biology: (i) to describe a group of individuals in terms of the group's own attributes and qualities; (ii) to measure the precision of an estimate with high confidence; (iii) to measure the degree of association between the variations in a series of characters or events (see [46]). These three fundamental methods are discussed at length in the present textbook.

Biostatistics is an interdisciplinary subject which lies at the intersection of biology and statistics, and consists in the study of quantitative or statistical methods applied to biology. This subject has a recent history, its origins dating back to Francis Galton, a cousin of Charles Darwin, who was interested in the problem of heredity. He used quantitative techniques (such as fitting a line to describe the association between two variables), to answer biological questions.

The field of biostatistics (also known as biometrics) was born in the late 19th century and early 20th century, mostly out of the work of Karl Pearson (the founder of the world's first statistics department at University College London) and Ronald Fisher (a pioneer in the field of experimental design). Both Pearson and Fisher developed statistical methods to answer questions from the biological sciences. In fact, the work of Gregor Mendel went unnoticed for many years by biologists, since they were not used to think in quantitative or statistical terms. It was Pearson and his peers that rediscovered Mendel's work, and the laws of inheritance.

The purpose of this book is to introduce the biology students to statistical reasoning and modeling, which are of critical importance to the foundations of modern biology.

Ottawa, February 15, 2011

Contents

PART 1
Probability

Chapter 1

Introduction to Probability

Probability theory was developed in the 17th century, from the study of games of chance by some French mathematicians, like Blaise Pascal and Pierre de Fermat. It was not until the 20th century that people realize that probability theory has deep connections with statistics, and can be used as an explanation for the variability exhibited by data sets. The underlying assumption is that the same unknown rules which make unpredictable the result of a game of chance can be used for explaining the nature of this variability. These rules have to do with the common underlying concept of randomness. In this chapter, we explain the concept of randomness and examine several methods for assigning probabilities to events.

1.1 Interpreting Probabilities

Statements about probabilities associated to various events are frequently encountered in everyday life. For instance, when predicting the weather, the news channels report the chances that a certain event (like rain) will take place; before the election date, the possible outcomes of the election are reported as percentages which represent the chances of winning for each candidate. Some events could be perceived as more likely than others due to the lack of proper information: since plane crashes are more often included in the news than car accidents, one may be tempted to think that motor vehicles are a safer mode of transportation than aircrafts.

It has become common knowledge that events which are unlikely to occur are associated with small probabilities, and events which are very likely to occur are associated with large probabilities. However, when dealing with random events, it is important to realize that the fact that an event has a small probability does not mean that this event cannot occur. A blackout like the one of August 14, 2003, which left 55 million people in Ontario and the Northeastern part of the United States without power, was considered an unlikely event, until it happened.

In general, probabilities are associated only with events which arise in situations when one cannot say with 100% confidence what the outcome will be. For example, the outcome of a surgery varies from patient to patient, and a surgeon cannot guarantee that the operation will be successful for all the patients. The outcome in such situations is subject to randomness.

Definition 1.1. We say that a **random experiment** is an experiment whose outcome is determined by chance and cannot be predicted with 100% accuracy. The set S of all possible outcomes of a random experiment is called the **sample space**. An **event** is a subset of S.

A classical example of a random experiment is flipping a coin. In this case, there are only two possible outcomes: the coin lands on heads, or tails. A medical operation can also be viewed as a random experiment, which has several possible outcomes: the patient could recover entirely, suffer side effects, need a second operation, or even die.

Definition 1.2. The **probability** of an event is a number between 0 and 1 (or a percentage), which represents the chance that the event will occur.

For instance, a dental surgeon estimates that the probability that a patient recovers entirely after a wisdom tooth removal is 99.9%.

There are three methods for assigning probabilities to events:

1. The personal method

When using this method, the probability represents a person's degree of belief that the event will take place. This is a subjective method, because it depends on the person's access to relevant information, and ability to assess the situation. It is the method that we use in real life when we are faced with situations that we encounter only rarely.

For instance, a student has an idea about the probability that she will have at least one job offer, after a series of interviews for a summer internship position. Without a map, a group of tourists can easily get lost in the Algonquin Park, and come up with different probabilities for the event that a certain path will take them back to the camp site.

The problem with the personal method is that it does not have a scientific basis, and therefore it is not accurate. It is certainly not the method that will be used in this book. We mention it because of its wide applicability.

2. The relative frequency method

To use this method, the random experiment has to be repeated a large number of times. If in a sequence of n repetitions of the experiment, the event A occurs f times, then the probability of A is defined as:

$$P(A) = \frac{f}{n}.$$

Example 1.1. In the study [11] regarding the injuries associated with the use of Tasers (weapons that use electrical current), among the 1,000 cases examined, 997 persons had mild injuries, and 3 persons had serious injuries and needed hospitalization. The probability that a person will have serious injuries after being shot by a Taser is $3/1,000 = 0.003$.

Example 1.2. A neurologist noticed that among the 565 cases of epileptic children who received a low dose of anti-epileptic medication, 32 reported side effects to the medication. He concludes that the probability that this medication will have side effects in children even when used in a low dose is $32/565 = 0.057$.

The relative frequency method is more accurate than the personal method, but requires some prior information about the frequencies associated with the outcomes of the random experiment. The larger the number n of repetitions, the more accurate the probability of the event A will be.

3. The classical method

This method is used when the random experiment has a finite number of equally likely outcomes. We denote by $n(S)$ the number of elements in S. An event A can be regarded as a subset of S, which contains $n(A)$ elements. The probability of the event A is defined as:

$$P(A) = \frac{n(A)}{n(S)}$$

Example 1.3. An animal shelter has received a litter of 5 kittens, which consists of 3 males and 2 females. One of them is randomly selected for adoption. Since the 5 kittens are equally likely to be selected, and 2 of them are females, the probability that the chosen kitten is a female is $2/5 = 0.4$.

The classical method is very accurate, and can be used in a variety of situations. These include examples from genetics that will be examined in the next chapter.

Did you know that? *Louis Pasteur was born in France in 1822 and grew up during a period in which the French society underwent deep modernization. Despite this, the medical treatment in the first half of the 19th century was still closed to the medieval practices. At 32, as a young chemist and the newly appointed dean of the Faculty of Sciences in Lille, Pasteur was about to change this forever. Combining patient observations with the use of experimental methods, over the course of two decades, he developed the germ theory of disease, which became slowly accepted by the younger generation of doctors. His experiments marked the beginning of microbiology, the scientific study of microscopic forms of life. An interesting episode happened during his experiments with the cholera microbe. On one of the rare occasions that Pasteur went on vacation, his two assistants Pierre Roux and Charles Chamberland decided to take a holiday too, leaving the cholera cultures unattended. When Pasteur returned and found the sterile cultures, he had a flash of inspiration. By inoculating the sterile cultures to a sample of chicken, he discovered that these chicken became immune to the cholera microbe. Pasteur postulated that the sterile cultures acted as a vaccine, and developed a theory of immunization. To convince the general public about the validity of his theory, he performed a public demonstration on May 5, 1881, in which 25 sheep and 5 cows were inoculated with the anthrax virus. It could be argued that this important discovery was made by chance. But, as Pasteur said in 1854, "in the field of observation, chance favors only the prepared mind". Due to his hard work, Pasteur was prepared to grasp this opportunity, offered to him by chance. Other interesting stories about scientific discoveries made by chance can be found in* [8].

Chapter 2

Elementary Genetics and Probability

In this chapter we explore the connections between the elementary theory of genetics and two important areas of mathematics, probability and combinatorics. Probability allows us to calculate the chances associated with the inheritance of certain genes, while combinatorics provides us with the tools which are necessary for evaluating the number of possible combinations of various genes.

2.1 Tree Diagrams and Punnett Squares

Initiated by Gregor Mendel's 1865 landmark paper, genetics is one of the areas where probability plays a crucial role. Mendel was the first who recognized the significance of statistical thinking in predicting the inheritance of certain traits. His quantitative methods of counting large number of pea plants with specific traits over several generations provided the basis for the law of segregation, without which the modern theory of genetics would not exist. In this section, we review Mendel's laws, and their connections with probability, as explained in [27].

Example 2.1 (Mendel's Example). Mendel began with purebred strains of peas, i.e. strains that were bred only with themselves for many generations. He crossed purebred yellow-seeded with purebred green-seeded plants. Though the peas resulting from this cross (called the F_1 generation) might have been a mixture between yellow and green, they all turned out to be yellow. Mendel then planted the F_1 seeds and crossed the resulting plants with one another to make a second generation F_2. Remarkably, some of the F_2 seeds were yellow, but some were green, with the green/yellow ratio close to 1/3: he obtained 2,001 green seeds and 6,022 yellow seeds in F_2. The other features Mendel studied showed the same pattern: in following the flower color, he obtained 224 white plants and 705 purple plants in F_2.

Mendel postulated that:

(i) Plants carry factors that determine the inheritance of each character (e.g. seed color).
(ii) Each plant carries a pair of hereditary factors for each character, one factor derived from each of its parents.
(iii) When a plant has two different factors, one of them is *dominant* (i.e. its effect is visible) while the other is *recessive* (i.e. its effect is hidden).

Today we recognize that Mendel's two factors are forms of a single gene that determines the character, and we call them *alleles* of each other. When both factors are the same, we say that the individual is *homozygous*; when the two factors are different, the individual is *heterozygous*.

A specification of the genes that an individual carries is called the *genotype*. The expressed character of an individual is called the *phenotype*.

The major breakthrough of Mendel's discovery (which became later a solid base for explaining Darwin's theory of evolution by natural selection), can be summarized as follows: *An organism can carry a genetic potential that it does not exhibit!*

Example 2.1 (Continued). Mendel's explanation for his results was the following. Yellow seed color is dominant, while green seed color is recessive. The purebred yellow seed carries two Y factors (YY), and the purebred green seed carries two y factors (yy). These plants are homozygous. Since the original plants contribute one factor for seed color, all the F_1 plants are Yy, i.e they are heterozygous. Each plant in the F_1 generation produces two types of gametes: half of them carry Y, and half carry y. (The fact that the two genes segregate from each other, so that each gamete contains only one of them is called "the law of segregation".) These gametes combine at random to produce one of the 4 combinations: YY, Yy, yY or yy. Among these 4 combinations, 1 yields green seeds (yy), and 3 yield yellow seeds (YY, Yy, yY). This explains the observed green/yellow ratio close to 1/3.

This experiment can be illustrated using a *Punnett square* (see Figure 2.1) or a *tree diagram* (see Figure 2.2).

Female Gamete	Male Gamete $\frac{1}{2}Y$	Male Gamete $\frac{1}{2}y$
$\frac{1}{2}Y$	$\frac{1}{4}YY$ (yellow)	$\frac{1}{4}Yy$ (yellow)
$\frac{1}{2}y$	$\frac{1}{4}yY$ (yellow)	$\frac{1}{4}yy$ (green)

Fig. 2.1 Punnett square for Mendel's experiment

Female Gamete	Male Gamete	Offspring Genotype	Offspring Phenotype	Probability
Y	Y	YY	yellow	1/4
	y	Yy	yellow	1/4
y	Y	yY	yellow	1/4
	y	yy	green	1/4

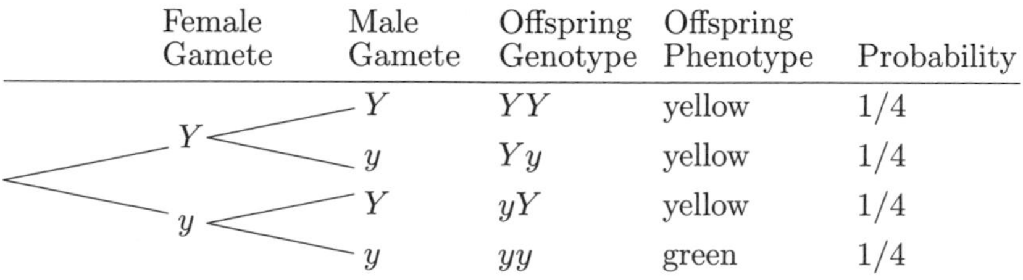

Fig. 2.2 Tree diagram for Mendel's experiment

Note that this diagram corresponds to the familiar chance operation of flipping two coins, in which case the 4 equally probable outcomes are HH, HT, TH, TT, where H =head and T = tail. Similarly, we can use the same diagram for determining the children's sex in a family with 2 children: the 4 outcomes are MM, MF, FM, FF, where M =male and F = female.

In general, many simple examples in genetics, dealing with equally likely outcomes, can be represented using the tree diagram method. The idea is simple: start with a common "root" and then draw one branch of the tree for each possible outcome.

Example 2.2. This example examines the genetics of the A-B-O blood system. Type A people have only A antigens on their blood cells and have antibodies in their serum against type B blood cells. The opposite is true for type B. Type AB people have both A and B antigens on their blood cells. Type O people have neither A nor B antigens. The blood type is determined by three alleles of a gene denoted by I. (This is an example of a gene with multiple alleles.) The allele I^A determines type A antigens, I^B determines type B antigens, and i specifies no antigen at all. I^A and I^B

are dominant over i, but I^A and I^B are codominant with each other, i.e.
(a) a type A person can have genotype I^AI^A or I^Ai,
(b) a type B person can have genotype I^BI^B or I^Bi,
(c) a type O person has genotype ii,
(d) a type AB person has genotype I^AI^B.

A woman has type A blood and is heterozygous; hence, her genotype is I^Ai. A man has type AB blood; hence, his genotype is I^AI^B. To determine the genotype of their child, we cross $I^Ai \times I^AI^B$. We use the Punnett square (see Figure 2.3) to illustrate the possible genotypes for the offspring, and the associated probabilities. The phenotypes are between the parenthesis. The child can have type A blood with probability 1/2, type B blood with

Female Gamete	Male Gamete $\frac{1}{2}I^A$	$\frac{1}{2}I^B$
$\frac{1}{2}I^A$	$\frac{1}{4}I^AI^A$ (type A)	$\frac{1}{4}I^AI^B$ (type AB)
$\frac{1}{2}i$	$\frac{1}{4}iI^A$ (type A)	$\frac{1}{4}iI^B$ (type B)

Fig. 2.3 Punnett square for $I^Ai \times I^AI^B$

probability 1/4, and type AB blood with probability 1/4. Note that in this case, the child cannot have type O blood: the probability that the child has type O blood is 0. For this reason, blood types can sometimes be used in cases of disputed paternity. The same conclusion can be reached using the tree diagram (see Figure 2.4)

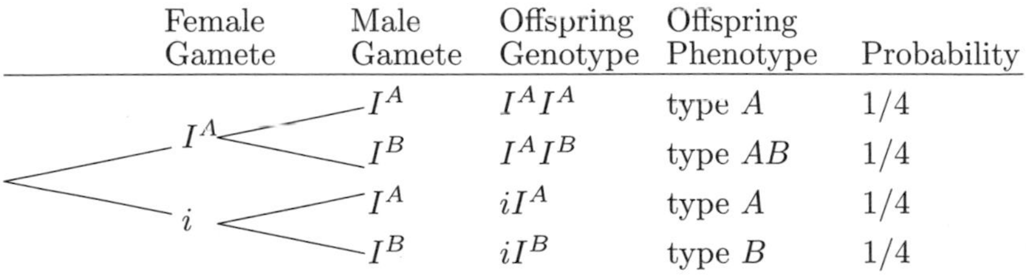

Female Gamete	Male Gamete	Offspring Genotype	Offspring Phenotype	Probability
I^A	I^A	I^AI^A	type A	1/4
	I^B	I^AI^B	type AB	1/4
i	I^A	iI^A	type A	1/4
	I^B	iI^B	type B	1/4

Fig. 2.4 Tree diagram for $I^Ai \times I^AI^B$

Sometimes, two or more genes are considered simultaneously. Mendel performed such experiments in which he considered two characters together (e.g. seed color and seed shape), and observed that the two alleles of the two genes assort independently when gametes are formed. This is called "the law of independent assortment".

Example 2.3. In humans, the hair color is determined by a gene whose allele for dark hair (D) is dominant over the allele for red hair (d), while the eye color is determined by a gene whose allele for brown eyes (B) is dominant over the allele for blue eyes (b). A women is red-haired and has blue eyes; hence, her genotype is $ddbb$. A man is dark-haired and has brown eyes, but he is heterozygous for both genes, i.e. his genotype is $DdBb$.

To calculate the probability that their child is red-haired and has blue eyes, we draw the Punnett square (see Figure 2.5) which gives all the possible genotypes and phenotypes for their child.

Female Gamete	Male Gamete			
	$\frac{1}{4}DB$	$\frac{1}{4}Db$	$\frac{1}{4}dB$	$\frac{1}{4}db$
db	$\frac{1}{4}dD\ bB$ (dark hair, brown eyes)	$\frac{1}{4}dD\ bb$ (dark hair, blue eyes)	$\frac{1}{4}dd\ bB$ (red hair, brown eyes)	$\frac{1}{4}dd\ bb$ (red hair, blue eyes)

Fig. 2.5 Punnett square for $ddbb \times DdBb$

The 4 possible genotypes for the children are: $dDbB$, $dDbb$, $ddbB$ and $ddbb$. These are equally probable. Among these, only one corresponds to a red-haired child with blue eyes ($ddbb$). Hence, the probability of a red-haired child with blue eyes is $1/4$. This can be illustrated by a tree diagram (see Figure 2.6).

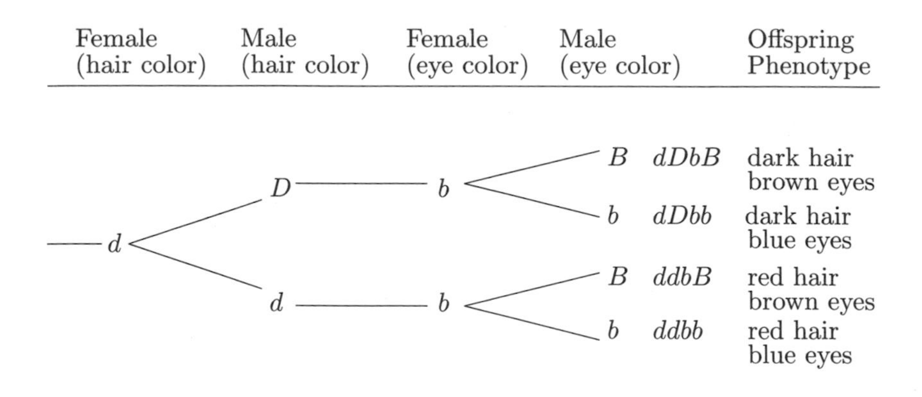

Fig. 2.6 Tree diagram for $ddbb \times DdBb$

2.2 Computation Methods

In Section 1.1, we saw that if the outcomes of an experiment are equally likely to occur, then the probability of an event A is calculated by the formula:

$$P(A) = \frac{n(A)}{n(S)}$$

where $n(A)$ denotes the number of possible ways in which the event A can occur, and $n(S)$ denotes the total number of outcomes of the experiment. If the experiment is rather simple and the total number of outcomes is not too large, then one can use the tree diagram method to compute the numbers $n(A)$ and $n(S)$. If the experiment is more complex, one has to consider specific methods for calculating $n(A)$ and $n(S)$. These methods are discussed in the present section.

Arrangement of objects in which the order is important are routinely encountered in everyday life: bank PIN numbers, telephone numbers, licence plate numbers, social insurance numbers, computer passwords, locker combinations, etc. As we see from these examples, the objects can be of different type: digits, letters, keyboard characters, etc. What matters is their order.

Example 2.4. To count the number of distinct 4-digit bank PIN numbers, we consider the operation of choosing each digit as a separate stage of the counting procedure; in this case, there are 4 stages. Next, we count how many possible choices are for each stage: there are 10 possible choices for the first digit (Stage 1), since this digit can be selected arbitrarily among the digits $0, 1, 2, \ldots, 9$; there are also 10 possible choices for the second digit (Stage 2), third digit (Stage 3), and fourth digit (Stage 4). Finally, we multiply the numbers obtained in Stages 1 to 4. We obtain $10 \cdot 10 \cdot 10 \cdot 10 = 10,000$ as the total number of 4-digit bank PIN numbers. Suppose now that someone finds a bank card and tries to use it by choosing at random a 4-digit number for its PIN. We want to find the probability that he will guess the correct number. In this case, S has $10,000$ possible outcomes, and the event A (consisting of the correct PIN selection) has only one outcome. Hence, $n(S) = 10,000$, $n(A) = 1$ and

$$P(A) = \frac{n(A)}{n(S)} = \frac{1}{10,000} = 0.0001.$$

Hence, the probability that he will guess the correct PIN number is 0.0001.

The rule used in the previous example is a useful procedure for computation purposes. It is called *the multiplication principle.* In summary, it relies on the following steps:

Step 1. Divide the experiment into stages 1, 2, 3, etc.
Step 2. Count how many possible choices are for each stage.
Step 3. Multiply the numbers obtained in *Step 2.*

Example 2.5. (a) To count the number of different 7-digit telephone numbers, which do not start with 0 or 1, we divide the counting procedure in 7 stages. The number of possible outcomes per stage are: $8, 10, 10, 10, 10, 10, 10$. By the multiplication principle, there are $8 \cdot 10^6 = 8,000,000$ telephone numbers.

(b) We want to see how many licence tags can be formed, which contain 4 letters and 3 digits. This counting procedure has 7 stages, whose number of possible outcomes are: $26, 26, 26, 26$ (for letters) and $10, 10, 10$ (for digits). The total number of license tags is $26^4 \cdot 10^3 = 456,976,000$. On the other hand, the number of license tags, which contain no repeated digits is $26^4 \cdot 10 \cdot 9 \cdot 8 = 329,022,720$. Since the digits must be distinct, the number of possible choices decreases by 1 for the last 3 stages.

The multiplication principle is frequently used in genetics. To illustrate its application in this context, we need to introduce some background material from biology. Most of this material is borrowed from [27].

It is known that *proteins* lie at the heart of all phenomena associated with life, each of them having a structure that is good for a different function. From the chemical point of view, a protein is a polymer made by linking different kinds of monomers called *amino acids*, which can be arranged in any sequence. An amino acid molecule contains one central carbon C atom linked to a hydrogen H atom, an amino NH_2 group, an organic acid $COOH$ group, and a side chain. The 20 existing amino acids differ only in the structure of their side chains. (Two amino acids can be linked by joining the $COOH$ group of the first with the NH_2 group of the next, with the removal of one molecule of water.) A sequence of 2, 3, or 4 amino acids is called a dipeptide, a tripeptide, or a tetrapeptide, respectively. A typical protein may have up to 300 amino acids joined in a single chain.

Example 2.6. By the multiplication principle, there are $20 \cdot 20 = 400$ dipeptides, $20^3 = 8,000$ tripetides, and $20^4 = 160,000$ tetrapeptides. There are 20^{300} different ways of making a chain of 300 amino acids. This number is larger than the number of proteins that ever existed on Earth. So, many of these combinations are not proteins. (Recent work on the human genome gives a range of 30,000-50,000 for the different proteins of the human body.)

Since a living organism consists of thousands of different proteins, its cells need specific information about how to line up the correct amino acids to make each of these proteins. This information lies in the deoxyribonucleic acid (DNA) and the ribonucleic acid (RNA). These are another kind of polymers, quite different from proteins, which consist of monomers, called *nucleotides*, that can be arranged in any sequence. A nucleotide has 3 parts: a base, linked to a sugar, which is linked to a phosphate (PO_4). DNA nucleotides have one of 4 bases: adenine (A), guanine (G), cytosine (C), thymine (T). In RNA, uracil (U) replaces thymine.

A DNA molecule carries information in the sequence of its monomers, and a cell uses this information to direct the synthesis of its proteins. A segment of DNA that specifies the structure of a polypeptide is called a *gene*. The linear sequence of bases in DNA can be viewed as a series of 3-letter code words (or *codons*) that specify the linear sequence of amino acids in proteins. Since DNA and protein are both linear molecules, the two sequences are *colinear.*

The DNA is located on a string-like structure (called chromosome) in the nucleus of the cell, but the protein is manufactured in the cytoplasm of the cell. The role of RNA is to carry the information from DNA to the cytoplasm: the RNA contains a series of codons copied from the DNA, in which U replaces T.

Example 2.7. By the multiplication principle, there are $4 \cdot 4 \cdot 4 = 64$ codons. It is known that of the 64 codons, 61 code for the 20 amino acids, and 3 are "stops" (i.e. they signal the end of a polypeptide chain). If a codon is chosen at random, the probability that it will code for an amino acid is:

$$P(A) = \frac{61}{64} = 0.953.$$

Consider the RNA segment $AAUUUGAUG$. This segment is formed of the following 3 codons: AAU (code for *asparagine*, or *asn*), UUG (code for *leucine*, or *leu*), AUG (code for *methionine*, or *met*), and hence it corresponds to the amino acid sequence *asn-leu-met*. There are 2 codes for asparagine (AAU and AAC), 6 codes for leucine (UUA, UUG, CUU, CUC, CUA, CUG) and 1 code for methionine. By the multiplication principle, there are $2 \cdot 6 \cdot 1 = 12$ codes for *asn-leu-met*.

In the previous example, the tripeptide *asn-leu-met* is different from *leu-asn-met*, which is obtained by exchanging the places of the first two amino acids. In fact, the 3 amino acids (*leu*, *asn*, *met*) can be arranged in 6 ways, leading to different tripeptides: by the multiplication principle, there are 3 ways of choosing the first amino acid, 2 ways of choosing the second one, and 1 way of choosing the third one; hence, the number of possible arrangements is $3 \cdot 2 \cdot 1 = 6$. These 6 arrangements are: *asn-leu-met*, *asn-met-leu*, *leu-asn-met*, *leu-met-asn*, *met-asn-leu*, *met-leu-asn*. They are called permutations of the 3 amino acids: *asn*, *leu*, *met*. In general, we have the following definition.

Definition 2.1. A **permutation** is an arrangement of n objects into a sequence with n positions, without any repetitions.

By the multiplication principle, the number of permutations of n objects is:

$$n \cdot (n-1) \cdot (n-2) \cdot \ldots \cdot 3 \cdot 2 \cdot 1 =: n!\ .$$

This number is called n *factorial.*

Example 2.8. A 7-codon RNA sequence is to be formed, containing 3 times ACU (code for *threonine*, or *thr*) and 4 times GGU (code for *glycine*, or *gly*). How many RNA sequences with this composition can be found?

First, we assign a label from 1 to 4 to the ACU codes, and a label from 1 to 3 to the GGU codes, i.e. we introduce a way of distinguishing the four

ACU codons and the three GGU codons from each other. This leads us to 7 objects:

$$[ACU]_1, [ACU]_2, [ACU]_3, [ACU]_4, [GGU]_1, [GGU]_2, [GGU]_3.$$

As we noted above, these 7 objects can be permuted in $7! = 5,040$ ways. Consider one of them, say:

$$[ACU]_4\ [ACU]_2\ [GGU]_3\ [ACU]_3\ [GGU]_2\ [ACU]_1\ [GGU]_1.$$

We now permute the ACU codons among themselves: any permutation will lead to the same RNA sequence, which has an ACU codon on positions 1, 2, 4 and 6 as above. (Since the labels were introduced artificially, they do not appear in the RNA sequence.) This gives us $4! = 24$ possible arrangements. Similarly, we permute the GGU's among themselves, and we obtain $3! = 6$ possible arrangements which have the GGU codons on positions 3, 5 and 7. By the multiplication principle, there are $24 \cdot 6 = 144$ different arrangements of the form $[ACU][ACU][GGU][ACU][GGU][ACU][GGU]$. These 144 sequences cannot be distinguished from each other, in the original collection of 5,040 arrangements (with labels). Therefore the 144 sequences have to be counted only once. The same argument applies to any one of the 5,040 arrangements (with labels). In other words, the 5,040 arrangements can be divided into groups consisting of 144 arrangements each, which become identical when we remove the labels. The number of such groups coincides with the number of RNA sequences, and is equal to $5,040/144 = 35$.

A different type of computation technique is needed when one selects a sample from a group of individuals. If the group consists of 4 persons, and we are interested in selecting 1 individual, then there are 4 possible choices. Suppose now that we are interested in selecting 2 individuals. By the multiplication principle, there are 4 ways of choosing the first person, and 3 ways of choosing the second one. This gives us $4 \cdot 3 = 12$ ways of choosing a pair of individuals, if their order is important. In our case, the order between the two individuals is not important. Since there are $2! = 2$ ways of permuting the 2 individuals, the total number of ways of selecting 2 individuals from a group of 4 is $12/2 = 6$. If the individuals are called A, B, C, D, one can easily list the 6 possible choices: $\{A, B\}$, $\{A, C\}$, $\{A, D\}$, $\{B, C\}$, $\{B, D\}$, $\{C, D\}$.

The following definition introduces the general concept.

Definition 2.2. A **combination** is a selection of objects from a group, in which the order is not important.

In general, the number of combinations of r objects selected from a group of n objects is given by the formula:

$$\frac{n \cdot (n-1) \cdot (n-2) \cdot \ldots \cdot (n-r+1)}{r!} =: \binom{n}{r}.$$

This number is called *n choose r*.

Examples of combinations from real life include: samples from a population, 13-card hands dealt from a 52-card deck, tickets at the 6/49 lottery, etc. (Note that a locker "combination" is in fact a permutation, since the order of the digits matters.)

Example 2.9. Ten patients are participating in a medical study. Among those, 4 have to be chosen for a new drug treatment. The number of possible selections is

$$\binom{10}{4} = \frac{10 \cdot 9 \cdot 8 \cdot 7}{4!} = \frac{5,040}{24} = 210.$$

Suppose now that 2 of the 10 patients are allergic to some compound found in the drug. We would like to see what is the probability that the group of 4 (randomly selected) patients includes at least one allergy case.

Let A be the event that the selected group does not include an allergy case. Since there are exactly

$$\binom{8}{4} = \frac{8 \cdot 7 \cdot 6 \cdot 5}{4!} = \frac{1,680}{24} = 70$$

ways of selecting the 4 patients among the 8 non-allergy cases, the number of possible ways event A can be realized is $n(A) = 70$. The probability of A is:

$$P(A) = \frac{n(A)}{n(S)} = \frac{70}{210} = \frac{1}{3}.$$

The probability of A', the event that A fails (i.e. the selection includes at least one allergy case) is:

$$P(A') = \frac{n(A')}{n(S)} = \frac{140}{210} = \frac{2}{3}.$$

(We used the fact that $n(A') = n(S) - n(A) = 210 - 70 = 140$.)

We now would like to find the probability of the event B that the group of 4 patients includes exactly one allergy case. Note that there are 2 ways of selecting one patient among the 2 allergy cases, and

$$\binom{8}{3} = \frac{8 \cdot 7 \cdot 6}{3!} = \frac{336}{6} = 56$$

ways of selecting the 3 remaining patients among the 8 non-allergy cases. By the multiplication principle, $n(B) = 2 \cdot 56 = 112$. The probability of B is:

$$P(B) = \frac{n(B)}{n(S)} = \frac{112}{210} = 0.533.$$

2.3 Problems

Problem 2.1. Rabbits injected with human blood cells develop antibodies against antigens on the human cells. These antibodies help identify two types of antigens, called M and N. Cells from a person with type M blood induce the rabbits to make anti-M antibodies. Cells from a person with type N blood induce the rabbits to make anti-N antibodies. Every person has blood of type M, type N, or type MN (which contains both antigens). The gene of this character is called L (in honor of Karl Landsteiner) and has two alleles denoted by L^M and L^N, which determine the type M and type N antigens, respectively. The two alleles are codominant. A person with type M blood has genotype $L^M L^M$; a person with type N blood has genotype $L^N L^N$; a person with type MN blood has genotype $L^M L^N$. Use a Punnett square or a tree diagram to illustrate all the possible genotypes and phenotypes of the offspring and the associated probabilities, in the following cases:
(a) the woman and the man have type MN blood;
(b) the woman has type M blood and the man has type MN blood;
(c) the woman has type M blood and the man has type N blood.

Problem 2.2. A chemical called phenylthiocarbamide (PTC) tastes very bitter to some people (tasters) but is tasteless to others (non-tasters). This character is hereditary, the taster allele (T) being dominant over the non-taster (t) allele. Another hereditary trait is albinism, the absence of pigments in skin, hair, and eyes. The gene determining skin pigmentation has two alleles: a dominant allele (A) for normal skin pigmentation, and a recessive allele (a) for albinism. Use a Punnett square or a tree diagram to illustrate all the possible genotypes and phenotypes of the offspring and the associated probabilities, in the following cases:
(a) the woman and the man are heterozygous for both genes;
(b) the woman is a heterozygous taster and an albino, and the man is a non-taster and is heterozygous with normal skin pigmentation;

(c) the woman is a non-taster and an albino, and the man is homozygous dominant for both genes.

In each case, calculate the probability of an albino non-taster offspring.

Problem 2.3. A group of 20 people consisting of 11 women and 9 men, has enrolled in a study about the factors which may influence the frequency and duration of migraines.
(a) The group has to be split into two subgroups of 10 persons each, for testing two different medications. In how many ways can this be done?
(b) At the end of the study, a sample of 10 persons has to be selected for filling out a questionnaire. The sample has to consist of 5 women and 5 men. In how many ways can the selection be done?
(c) The group consists of 8 smokers and 12 non-smokers. A sample of 8 persons is selected for participating in a drug-free migraine management program. What is the probability that the sample contains exactly 2 smokers?

Problem 2.4. The authors of [38] studied the frizzle character of fowls. A frizzled fowl has genotype FF, a normal fowl has genotype ff and a fowl with genotype Ff is slightly frizzled. This is an example of codominant alleles. Use the Punnett square or the tree diagram to illustrate all the possible genotypes and phenotypes of the offspring and the associated probabilities, in the following cases:
(a) both parents are slightly frizzled;
(b) only one parent is slightly frizzled and the other is normal;
(c) only one parent is slightly frizzled and the other is frizzled.

Problem 2.5. Epistasis is a process that explains how gene interaction can affect phenotypes (see [40]). Consider an example of epistasis which was explained by the authors of [18]. The colour of the flower of a pea plant can be purple or white, and is affected by two genes C and P which control the biochemistry of the plant. The flower is purple only if the dominant allele for both genes C and P are present.
(a) List all the possible genotypes for a pea plant with white flowers.
(b) Use the Punnett square or the tree diagram to illustrate all the possible genotypes and phenotypes (and the associated probabilities) of the offspring resulting from the cross of two pea plants with genotype $CcPp$. What is the probability that the offspring has purple flowers?

Problem 2.6. In a laboratory, a technician selects two samples from a

tray containing 15 samples. Assuming that among the 15 samples, four are tainted, what is the probability that the technician
(a) will select no tainted samples;
(b) will select exactly one tainted sample;
(c) will select two tainted samples.

Did you know that? *Gregor Johann Mendel was an Augustinian monk, who lived in Brünn, Austria (now Brno, Czech Republic), and had two interests outside the religious life: botany and statistics. He discovered the Mendelian laws of inheritance (which later led to the development of genetics) by patiently crossing pea plants in the monastery garden, and carefully recording the results. In 1865, he published his findings in a respectable (but rather obscure) journal called* Proceedings of the Natural History Society of Brünn. *Mendel died in 1884 without knowing the importance of his crucial discovery. In 1900, the same laws of inheritance were rediscovered independently by three other botanists: Hugo de Vries, Karl Correns, and Erich Tscermark. All three gave credit to Mendel, and published their work as a simple confirmation of a discovery made by an unknown monk decades ago. More details about this amazing story from the history of science can be found in* [6].

Chapter 3

Axioms of Probability

In the previous chapter, we were interested in calculating the probability of a single event A. In this chapter, we study some simple techniques which allow us to calculate the probabilities associated to two or more events which may occur simultaneously.

3.1 Venn Diagrams

The Venn diagram is a graphical method used in elementary set theory for representing subsets of a set S. This method is useful for illustrating situations in which we consider two or more events, each event A being regarded as a subset of the set S of all possible outcomes of a random experiment.

The idea is to represent the set S as a large rectangle, and a subset A as the region inside a closed curve in this rectangle. (The particular shape of the curve is not important.) This closed curve is called *the Venn diagram* of A.

We denote by A' the event that A fails, and we say that A' is *the complement* of A. Note that A' is represented by the region outside the same closed curve which is used for representing A.

Note that

$$1 = P(S) = P(A) + P(A'). \tag{3.1}$$

Example 3.1. A woman and a man are heterozygous for the gene which determines to eye color. Since the allele (B) for brown eyes is dominant over the allele (b) for blue eyes, both man and woman have genotype Bb. Similarly to Example 2.1, the offspring has a probability of $1/4$ of having blue eyes (i.e. the genotype bb), and a probability of $3/4$ of having brown

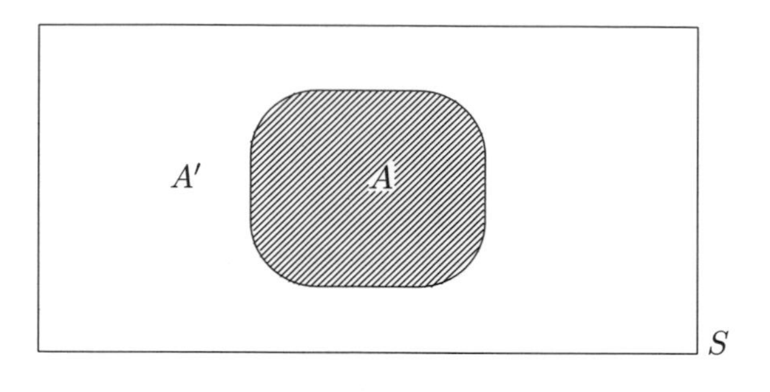

Fig. 3.1 The shaded region represents the event A

eyes (i.e. the genotype BB of Bb). Suppose that this couple has 3 children. We are interested in calculating the probability of the event A that they have at least one child with blue eyes.

The complement A' of A is the event that all 3 children have brown eyes. Hence

$$P(A') = \frac{3}{4} \cdot \frac{3}{4} \cdot \frac{3}{4} = \frac{27}{64}.$$

Using (3.1), it follows that:

$$P(A) = 1 - \frac{27}{64} = \frac{37}{64} = 0.578.$$

Let us consider two events A and B. We denote by $A \cap B$ the event that "A and B occur", and $A \cup B$ the event that "A or B occur". (The word "or" is understood in the non-exclusive sense, i.e. the possibility that A and B occur simultaneously is permitted in the event $A \cup B$.)

Suppose first that A and B cannot occur simultaneously. In this case, $A \cap B$ is the impossible event, denoted by $\emptyset$, and the events A and B are called *mutually exclusive*. The Venn diagrams of A and B are not overlapping.

We have:

$$P(A \cup B) = P(A) + P(B) \quad \text{if} \quad A \cap B = \emptyset.$$

The simplest example of mutually exclusive events are A and A'. Since $A \cup A' = S$, we say that A and A' form a partition of S.

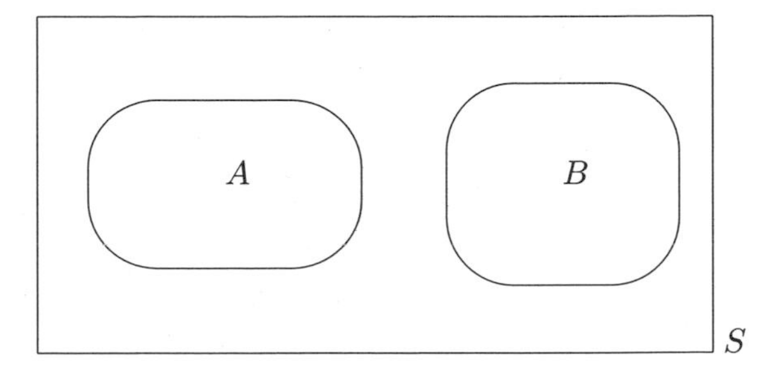

Fig. 3.2 The Venn diagrams of mutually exclusive events A and B

In general, we say that events $A_1, A_2, \ldots, A_k$ form a *partition* of S, if A_i and A_j are mutually exclusive for any $i \neq j$, and

$$A_1 \cup A_2 \cup \cdots \cup A_k = S.$$

Example 3.2. Among Canadians, 42% have type A blood, 9% have type B blood, 3% have type AB blood, and 46% have type O blood. A new patient is admitted into a hospital and needs a blood transfusion. We are interested in the event that this patient has blood of type A or type B.

We denote with A, B, C and D the events that the patient has the blood type A, B, AB, or O, respectively. These 4 events form a partition of S. To represent them, we draw the Venn diagrams of only 3 events (say A, B and C), using 3 non-overlapping curves, the region outside these curves representing the 4-th event.

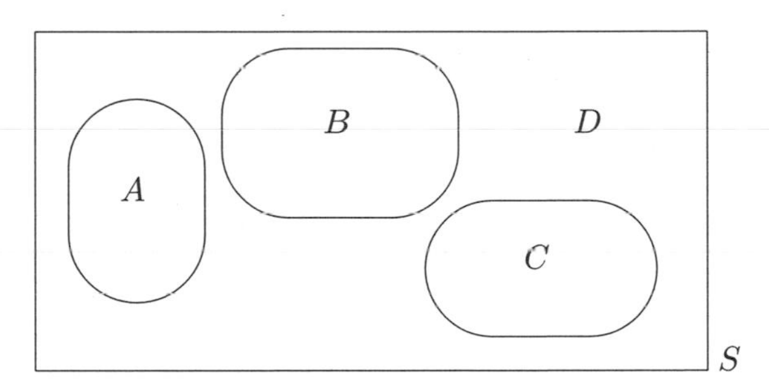

Fig. 3.3 Mutually exclusive events A, B, C, D, which form a partition of S

The desired probability is

$$P(A \cup B) = P(A) + P(B) = 0.42 + 0.09 = 0.51.$$

Note that the event $A \cup B$ is the complement of $C \cup D$. Since $P(C \cup D) = P(C) + P(D) = 0.03 + 0.46 = 0.49$, we could have argued also that

$$P(A \cup B) = 1 - P(C \cup D) = 1 - 0.49 = 0.51.$$

We consider now two events A and B which may occur simultaneously. In this case, the Venn diagrams representing A and B are overlapping (see Figure 3.4).

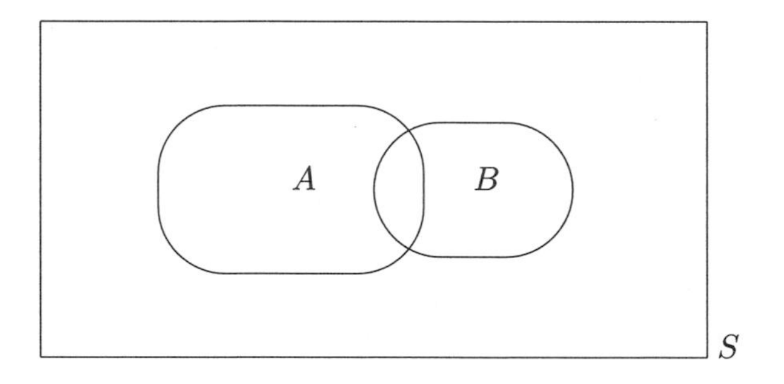

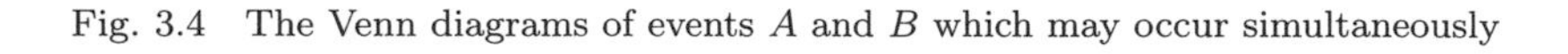

Fig. 3.4 The Venn diagrams of events A and B which may occur simultaneously

We distinguish several regions, which correspond to different events:

- The region in the middle represents the event $A \cap B$ (see Figure 3.5).

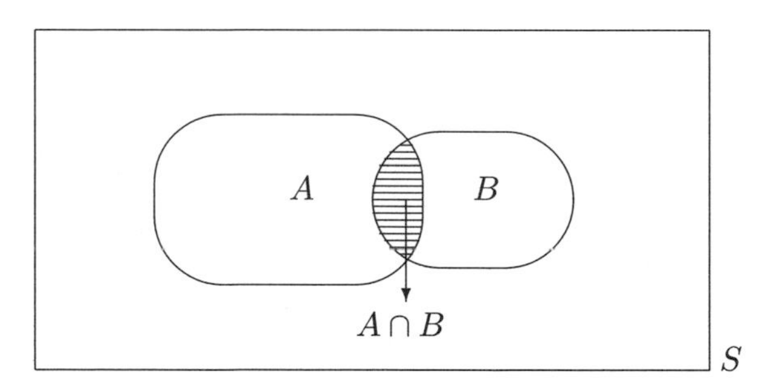

Fig. 3.5 The shaded region represents the event $A \cap B$

- The shaded region on the left represents the event "A occurs and B does not occur", denoted by $A \cap B'$ (see Figure 3.6). The probability of this event is linked to the probability of A by the following relation:

$$P(A) = P(A \cap B) + P(A \cap B').$$

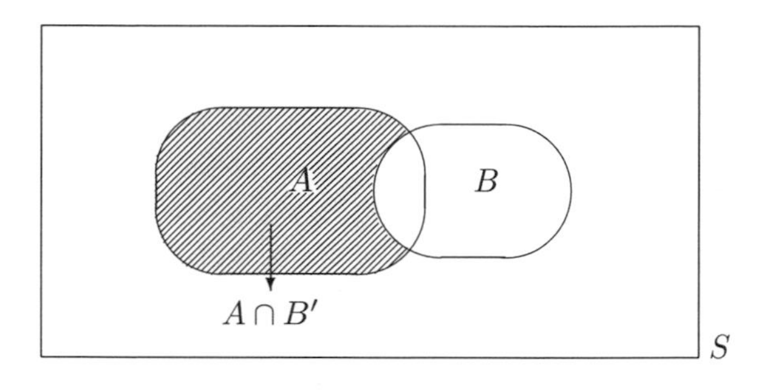

Fig. 3.6 The shaded region represents the event $A \cap B'$

Example 3.3. Consider a certain male population in which 48% are smokers, 5.5% have lung cancer and 4.9% are smokers with lung cancer. A random individual is selected from this population. Let A be the event that this individual is a smoker and B be the event that the individual has lung cancer. We know that $P(A) = 0.48$, $P(B) = 0.055$ and $P(A \cap B) = 0.049$.

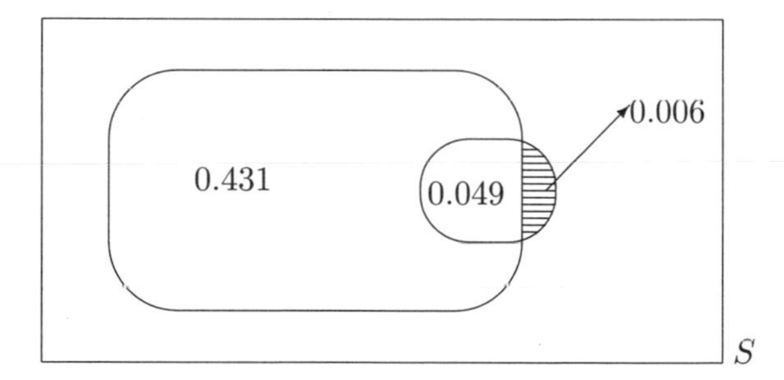

Fig. 3.7 The probabilities associated to the events $A \cap B'$, $A \cap B$ and $B' \cap A$

The probability that the randomly chosen individual is a smoker who does not have lung cancer is:

$$P(A \cap B') = P(A) - P(A \cap B) = 0.48 - 0.049 = 0.431.$$

The probability that the randomly chosen individual has lung cancer but is not a smoker is:

$$P(B \cap A') = P(B) - P(A \cap B) = 0.055 - 0.049 = 0.006.$$

Example 3.4. The percentage of people with diabetes in the Canadian aboriginal population is estimated to be higher than in the general population. A sample of 1,500 persons was randomly selected from the Canadian aboriginal population. Among these, 220 were diagnosed with diabetes and reported having a family physician, and 75 were diagnosed with diabetes, but reported not having a family physician. Calculate the probability that a randomly chosen Canadian aboriginal has diabetes.

Let A be the event the person has diabetes and B be the event that the person has a family physician. We know that $P(A \cap B) = 220/1,500$ and $P(A \cap B') = 75/1,500$. Hence.

$$P(A) = P(A \cap B) + P(A \cap B') = \frac{220 + 75}{1,500} = 0.197.$$

3.2 Addition Rule

When the events A and B are not mutually exclusive, the Venn diagram of the event $A \cup B$ is the closed curve obtained by joining the Venn diagrams of A and B. The region situated outside this curve corresponds to the complement of $A \cup B$, which is the event $A' \cap B'$.

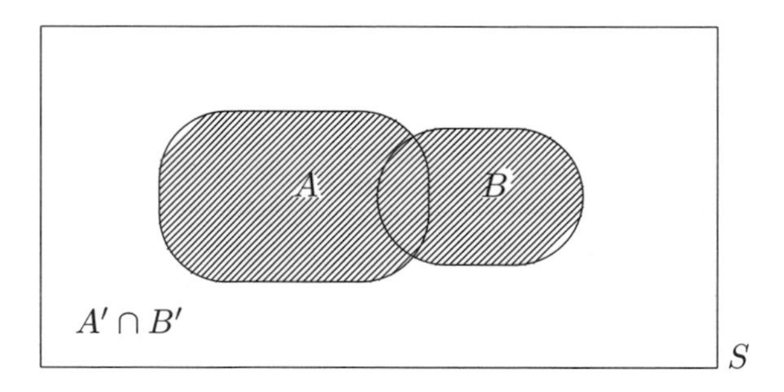

Fig. 3.8 The shaded region represents the event $A \cup B$

The probability of the event $A \cup B$ ("A or B occurs") can be calculated using the following *addition rule*:

$$P(A \cup B) = P(A) + P(B) - P(A \cap B). \tag{3.2}$$

To justify this rule, recall that the possibility that both A and B occur is permitted in our definition of the event $A \cup B$. Therefore, the event "A or B occurs" means

- either A and B occur simultaneously;
- or A occurs, but B does not occur;
- or B occurs, but A does not occur.

The three possibilities listed above correspond to the mutually exclusive events $A \cap B$, $A' \cap B$ and $B' \cap A$. These 3 events form a partition of $A \cup B$, and therefore:

$$P(A \cup B) = P(A \cap B) + P(A \cap B') + P(B \cap A'). \tag{3.3}$$

On the other hand, we have seen in Section 3.1 that

$$P(A) = P(A \cap B) + P(A \cap B')$$
$$P(B) = P(A \cap B) + P(B \cap A').$$

Taking the sum of the previous two equalities, we obtain:

$$P(A) + P(B) = 2P(A \cap B) + P(A \cap B') + P(B \cap A').$$

Subtracting $P(A \cap B)$ from both sides of this equality, we get:

$$P(A) + P(B) - P(A \cap B) = P(A \cap B) + P(A \cap B') + P(B \cap A'). \tag{3.4}$$

Relation (3.2) follows from (3.3) and (3.4).

Example 3.5. In sub-Sahara Africa, one child in three suffers from malnutrition. In the same region, one in five children are born HIV positive, due to the transmission from the mother to the newborn. Ten percent of the children population of this region suffers from both conditions.

A child is randomly selected from this population. We are interested in the probability that the child suffers from either one of these conditions.

Let A be the event that the child suffers from malnutrition and B be the event that the child is HIV positive. We know that

$$P(A) = \frac{1}{3}, \quad P(B) = \frac{1}{5}, \quad P(A \cap B) = \frac{1}{10}.$$

The probability that the child is malnourished or HIV positive is:

$$P(A \cup B) = P(A) + P(B) - P(A \cap B) = \frac{1}{3} + \frac{1}{5} - \frac{1}{10} = \frac{13}{30} = 0.433.$$

Note that the probability that the child suffers from neither one of these conditions is:

$$P(A' \cap B') = 1 - P(A \cup B) = 1 - 0.433 = 0.577.$$

The addition rule can also be used to calculate $P(A \cap B)$, since from (3.2), we deduce that

$$P(A \cap B) = P(A) + P(B) - P(A \cup B).$$

Note that the complement of $A \cap B$ is the event $A' \cup B'$, which says that "either A or B fails".

Example 3.6. The symptoms of the seasonal flu include fever (in 90% of the population), and muscular pain (in 80% of the population). When infected with the flu virus, 95% of the population has either one of the two symptoms.

We calculate the probability that a patient with the seasonal flu has both symptoms. Let A be the event that the patient has fever, and B be the event that the patient has muscular pain. We know that

$$P(A) = 0.90, \quad P(B) = 0.80, \quad P(A \cup B) = 0.95.$$

The desired probability is

$$P(A \cap B) = P(A) + P(B) - P(A \cup B) = 0.90 + 0.80 - 0.95 = 0.75.$$

3.3 Problems

Problem 3.1. Due to an inappropriate nutrition program, the chicken in a large poultry farm have developed some nutritional diseases. It is estimated that 2% of the poultry have the fatty liver syndrome, a condition characterized by obesity and an enlarged fatty liver, and 3% suffer from cage layer fatigue, a condition which results in soft bones, similar to osteoporosis. 4% of the chickens have either one of the conditions, but not both.
(a) Find the percentage of chicken which have both conditions.
(b) A chicken is randomly selected from this farm. What is the probability that it has neither one of the two conditions?

Problem 3.2. The official languages in Canada are English and French. Ottawa is a multicultural city whose residents have a diverse linguistic background. According to a 2006 Statistics Canada census, 59.9% of the residents of the city of Ottawa speak only English, 1.6% speak only French, and 1.3% speak neither one of the official languages.
(a) What is the percentage of the city of Ottawa residents who speak one of the official languages?
(b) What is the probability that a randomly chosen resident of the city of Ottawa speaks both official languages?

Problem 3.3. The Rideau Canal connects the Ottawa river with lake Ontario. In the winter, a section of 7.8 km of the canal which passes through the city of Ottawa is open for public skating, being the world's largest naturally frozen skating rink. Typically, it takes 10 to 14 days of continuous cold temperature (-15 degrees Celsius or colder) to form safe ice, which would allow the canal to be open for public skating. Meteorological data collected during the past 40 years shows that, during the 120 days of winter season, on average, the canal was open for public skating for 50 days, and the weather was sunny for 54 days. On average, a winter season would have 33 sunny days when the canal is open for public skating.
(a) What is the probability that on a randomly chosen day during the winter season, the canal is open for public skating, but the weather is not sunny?
(b) What is the probability that on a randomly chosen day during the winter season, the weather is sunny, but the canal is not open for public skating?

Problem 3.4. Consider a population of subjects such that 23% have a certain disease, 19% have been exposed to a certain risk factor, and 31% have been exposed to the risk factor or have the disease. What is the probability that a subject from this population
(a) has been exposed to the risk factor and has the disease?
(b) has been exposed to the risk factor, but does not have the disease?
(c) has the disease, but has not been exposed to the risk factor?

Problem 3.5. Consider 16 gallons of genetically modified tomatoes. Suppose that 75% of these tomatoes have an increased resistance to pests, 50% were engineered to have a longer shelf life, and 30% have an increased resistance to pests and were engineered to have a longer shelf life. If one of these tomatoes is randomly selected, compute the probability that this tomato
(a) has an increased resistance to pests, but was not engineered to have a longer shelf life;
(b) has an increased resistance to pests or was engineered to have a longer shelf life;
(c) does not have an increased resistance to pests, but was engineered to have a longer shelf life;
(d) does not have an increased resistance to pests and was not engineered to have a longer shelf life.

Problem 3.6. Some parents are permissive regarding the alcohol consumption and the cigarette use by their adolescent children. Assume that 13% of the parents permit the cigarette use in the house, 8.5% of the parents permit the alcohol consumption in the house, and 6% of the parents permit both cigarette use and alcohol consumption in the house. In a randomly chosen house, what is the probability that the parents permit:
(a) the use of at least one of the two substances;
(b) the cigarette use, but not the alcohol consumption;
(c) the consumption of alcohol, but not the cigarette use.

Did you know that? *In 2008, the Rideau Canal (a waterway located in Ontario, Canada) was declared a World Heritage Site by UNESCO (source: http://whc.unesco.org/en/list). It is a series of lakes and rivers stretching from Kingston in the south to Ottawa in the north, and connected by man-made canals and locks. The canal was opened in 1832 and the locks are still operating much as they were when it was first opened. The waterway spans a distance of 202 km. The Rideau Canal was build for military purposes, allowing the British forces to defend the colony of Canada against the United States of America. It is an alternate route from Lake Ontario to the St. Lawrence river that flows to the Atlantic Ocean. Lieutenant-Colonel John By (a British military engineer), the architect of the Rideau Canal, decided to create a slackwater canal system, flooding rapids rather than bypassing them with canal cuts. In doing so, he created many lake and marsh environments, home to hundreds of species of plants and animals (source: http://Rideau-Info.com). The greatest post-canal change took hold at the north end of the canal. The community thrived, became the City of Ottawa in 1855, and was chosen as the site of Canada's national capital by Queen Victoria in 1859. Every winter since 1971, the National Capital Commission (of Canada) maintains the ice surface of the Rideau Canal (in Ottawa), making it the largest skating rink in the world. The skateway spans a distance of 7.8 kilometers. It is a great way to see some of Ottawa's attractions, or quickly commute to work or school. In fact, both authors enjoy skating on the Rideau Canal to travel the 5 kilometers between the University of Ottawa and Carleton University (both universities are located in Ottawa, Ontario, Canada).*

Chapter 4

Conditional Probability

In this chapter we introduce the concept of conditional probability. Often we want to restrict the focus of the study or want to compute the probability of an event with access to partial information. In such cases we are interested in conditional probabilities. We will also see that conditional probabilities can be used as a tool to simplify the computation of a probability in some cases.

4.1 Definition

We motivate the concept of conditional probability by way of a few examples.

Example 4.1. In Ontario, legal fishing requires a fish to actively strike and bite on a hook. Hooking a fish anywhere else on the body is considered foul-hooking and the fish must be released. We are interested in the probability that an angler will unintentionally foul-hook a fish in a particular bay. Furthermore, we believe that the use of a jig instead of live bait might increase the chances of unintentional foul-hooking. During a fishing season we interview some randomly selected anglers. The data is presented in Table 4.1.

Table 4.1 Foul-hooking fish

	Foul hook		
fishing method	no foul	foul	total
jig	35	20	55
live bait	41	4	45
total	76	24	100

Using the relative frequency approach we can estimate the probability of foul-hooking a fish in this bay as $24/100 = 24\%$. Does the use of a jig affect this probability? We only consider the hooked fish with the condition that a jig had been used. Out of the 55 fish that were hooked with a jig, only 20 were foul-hooks. We estimate the probability of foul-hooking a fish in this bay, given that a jig is used, as $20/55 = 36.4\%$. It appears that the use of a jig will increase our chances of foul-hooking.

Example 4.2. The authors of [34] studied the germination of different species native to Australia. Germinability was expressed as a percentage of viable seeds that germinated after 10 days. Germination was defined as the time of emergence of an embryo through the seed coat. Some of the data is presented in Table 4.2.

Table 4.2 Germination of 95 different species

Germination Speed	Germinability Low	Intermediate	High	Total
Fast	14	4	4	22
Medium	36	22	2	60
Slow	6	13	4	23
Total	56	39	10	105

We can use these data as a probability model to describe the actual germination in Australia. We select a species at random and hence we can assume that each of the 105 species are equally likely. The probability that the species has high germinability is $P(A) = n(A)/n(S) = 10/105 = 0.095$, where $A =$"high germinability". Does the germination speed affect this probability? If we narrow our focus to species with a fast germination speed, then intuitively, the probability of high germinability should be $4/22 = 0.182$, since 4 of the 22 species in this class are classified as high. Within the event $B =$"fast germination speed", the probability that A will occur is

$$P(A|B) = \frac{4}{22} = \frac{n(A \cap B)}{n(B)} = \frac{n(A \cap B)/n(S)}{n(B)/n(S)} = \frac{P(A \cap B)}{P(B)}.$$

The preceding examples bring us to the following definition.

Definition 4.1. Let B be an event with $P(B) > 0$. The **conditional probability** of an event A, given that the event B has occurred is defined as

$$P(A|B) = \frac{P(A \cap B)}{P(B)}.$$

It is often useful to think of the statement "given the event B" as an indication that B plays the role of the sample space. Consider again Example 4.2. The probability of A ="high germinability" given C ="medium germination speed" is

$$P(A|C) = \frac{P(A \cap C)}{P(C)} = \frac{2/105}{60/105} = \frac{2}{60}.$$

For a fixed event B, it can be shown that the function $P(\cdot|B)$ is a probability function. For example, we can use the complement rule. If the probability of foul-hooking given the use of a jig is 0.364, then the probability of no foul-hooking given the use of a jig is $1 - 0.364 = 0.636$.

Example 4.3. The species *drosophila melanogaster* (also known as the fruit fly) is a commonly used model organism in biology classrooms. In the early 20th century Thomas Hunt Morgan described many mutations in drosophila (see [2]). For example, Morgan was the first to observe the white eye mutation in drosophila. The normal eye color is red.

We study a population of drosophila in which 25% of the flies have curly wings and 2% of the flies have purple eyes. Furthermore, 1% of the flies have both mutations. If we select a fly at random and this fly has curly wings, what is the probability that it also has purple eyes? Let E = "purple eye mutation" and W = "curly wing mutation", then the answer is the following conditional probability:

$$P(E|W) = \frac{P(E \cap W)}{P(W)} = \frac{0.01}{0.25} = 0.04.$$

Note that this probability is not equal to the proportion of the purple eyed flies that have curly wings, which is

$$P(W|E) = \frac{P(W \cap E)}{P(E)} = \frac{0.01}{0.02} = 0.5.$$

In the previous example we see that $P(A|B)$ is not equal to $P(B|A)$. As it is pointed out in [3], it is a common mistake of students to confuse the two probabilities. To avoid this mistake it is important to properly interpret the probability within the context of the problem. In Example 4.3, $P(W|E)$ is the proportion of the purple eyed flies that have curly wings, while $P(E|W)$ is the proportion of the curly winged flies that have purple eyes.

In the paragraphs that follow, we see that conditional probabilities are useful to assess the performance of diagnostic tests.

A diagnostic test is a tool that is used to assess the presence or absence of some condition. For example an enzyme immunoassay is often used as an initial screen for HIV detection. Hair analysis is another example of a diagnostic tool that is used in the fields of forensic toxicology, environmental toxicology and occupational health (see [41]).

A unit (called a subject if the unit is human) is said to be *positive* if it has the condition of interest, e.g. the subject has the disease. A *negative* unit means that the condition is absent. Most diagnostic tests are not perfect. The test result can be negative or positive. If the test result is positive but the unit is negative, then we say that it is a *false positive.* A *false negative* is a negative test result for a positive unit.

We can assess the performance of a diagnostic test with its sensitivity, specificity, positive predictive value and negative predictive value. In Table 4.3, a population of subjects are cross-classified according to the presence or absence of the condition, and also according to their test result.

Table 4.3 Results for a diagnostic test

	true condition	
test result	positive (U_+)	negative (U_-)
positive (T_+)	9.5%	1.8%
negative (T_-)	0.5%	88.2%

We consider a diagnostic test as *sensitive* if it is highly likely to react (i.e. give a positive result), when exposed to the appropriate stimulus (i.e. the unit is truly positive). We define the *sensitivity* of the diagnostic test as the conditional probability that a truly positive unit has a positive test result. In our example, the sensitivity is $P(T_+|U_+) = 9.5\%/(9.5\% + 0.5\%) = 95\%$. This means that 95% of the subjects with the disease have been correctly classified. The *false negative rate* is defined as $\beta = P(T_-|U_+) = 1 - P(T_+|U_+)$, which is 5% in our example. This means that 5% of the subjects with the disease have a negative test result.

A good diagnostic test has to be sensitive, but also *specific.* We do not want the test to be likely to react (i.e. give a positive result), when the condition is absent. We define the *specificity* of the diagnostic test as the conditional probability that a truly negative unit has a negative test result. In our example, the specificity is $P(T_-|U_-) = 88.2\%/(88.2\% + 1.8\%) = 98\%$. This means that 98% of the subjects without the disease are correctly classified. The *false positive rate* is defined as $\alpha = P(T_+|U_-) = 1 - P(T_-|U_-)$, which is 2% in our example. This means that 2% of the subjects without the disease have a positive test result.

A good diagnostic test has to be sensitive and specific. However, we still do not have the whole picture. Of most interest to the subject and the physician is his/her chances of having the disease given that the test result is positive, or his/her chances of not having the disease given that the test result is negative. The corresponding metrics are the *positive predictive value*, which is the probability that a unit that tests positive does have the condition and the *negative predictive value*, which is the probability that a unit that tests negative does not have the condition. In our example, the positive predictive value is $\mathsf{PPV} = P(U_+|T_+) = 9.5\%/(9.5\% + 1.8\%) = 84.1\%$ and the negative predictive value is $\mathsf{NPV} = P(U_-|T_-) = 88.2\%/(88.2\% + 0.5\%) = 99.4\%$.

4.2 Multiplication Rule

In some circumstances it might be easy to compute $P(A|B)$. If we also know $P(B)$, then we can use the definition of conditional probability and find $P(A \cap B)$. We get the following *multiplication rule*:

$$P(A \cap B) = P(A|B)P(B).$$

The multiplication rule is a technique of "conditioning". Above we are *conditioning* on the occurrence of the event B. However, we can also condition on the occurrence of the event A and obtain:

$$P(A \cap B) = P(B|A)P(A).$$

Example 4.4. People with Rh Negative blood of type O are considered universal donors because patients of all blood types can receive their blood. It is estimated that 46% of all Canadians have type O blood. Among these type O donors, about 15% are Rh Negative. We use the multiplication rule to determine the proportion of Canadians who have Rh Negative blood of type O. Define the events O and $Rh-$ as "type O blood" and "Rh negative", respectively. We know that $P(O) = 0.46$ and $P(Rh - |O) = 0.15$. Hence, the probability that a Canadian has both type O blood and is Rh negative is

$$\begin{aligned} P(O \cap Rh-) &= P(Rh - |O)P(O) \\ &= (0.15)(0.46) = 0.069 \quad \text{(or 6.9\%)}. \end{aligned}$$

Example 4.5. Surfactants (also known as "wetting agents") can be used on hydrophobic soil to allow water to penetrate and be absorbed. In particular, wetting agents are used by golf course superintendents for fighting localized dry spots.

To compare the effectiveness of a few surfactants, we assign randomly the surfactants to experimental units (i.e. soil samples). Suppose that there are 10 experimental units (labeled 1 through 10), and that we select randomly one at a time for the assignment. What is the probability that we will first choose unit 5, and then unit 4?

Let A be the event that unit 5 is chosen in the first selection, and B be the event that unit 4 is chosen in the second selection. If unit 5 was chosen first, then unit 4 is one possible result for the second selection among the 9 remaining units. Thus, it is reasonable to take $P(B|A) = 1/9$. By the multiplication rule, the probability that we will first choose unit 5 and then unit 4 is

$$P(A \cap B) = P(B|A)P(A) = \frac{1}{9} \cdot \frac{1}{10} = \frac{1}{90}.$$

Many processes of interest involve more than 2 events. The multiplication rule can be extended to three or more events as follows:

$$P(A_1 \cap \cdots \cap A_n) = P(A_1)P(A_2|A_1)P(A_3|A_1 \cap A_2) \cdots P(A_n|A_1 \cap \cdots \cap A_{n-1}).$$

Example 4.6. In the study of population health and risk assessments, we often select a sample of subjects from a target population. The sampling is carried out through stages. For example, our sampling scheme might involve selecting a few cities, then selecting a few streets from these cities, and then selecting one household from each of the selected streets.

Suppose that our household is one among ten on Bass Avenue, which is a street in the city of Pike. The investigators use a sampling design that selects the city of Pike with a probability of 20% and if the city of Pike is selected, then Bass Avenue is selected with a probability of 5%. What is the probability that our household is chosen to take part in the study? Since we are selected only if our household, street and city are selected simultaneously, the probability that our household is selected is

$$\begin{aligned} &P(\text{"Pike"})P(\text{"Bass"}|\text{"Pike"})P(\text{"our house"}|\text{"Bass"} \cap \text{"Pike"}) \\ &= (0.2)(0.05)(0.1) = 0.001. \end{aligned}$$

We end this section with a few examples that use a tree diagram to help us visualize conditional probabilities. To build the diagram think of the multiplication rule in steps. The tree diagram, in Figure 4.1 is an illustration of our application of the multiplication rule in Example 4.6.

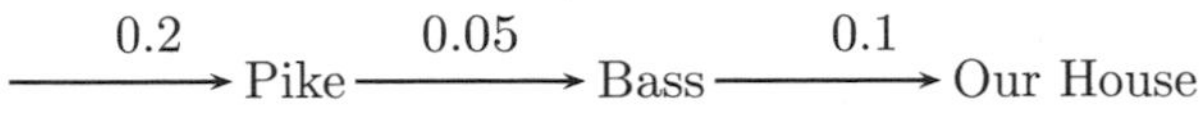

$$\xrightarrow{0.2} \text{Pike} \xrightarrow{0.05} \text{Bass} \xrightarrow{0.1} \text{Our House}$$

Fig. 4.1 Tree diagram: Visualizing the multiplication rule

Example 4.7. Beginning in the 1950s Kettlewell performed a series of experiments involving peppered moths (*Biston betularia*) in England (see [35]). Following the industrial revolution, the darker coloured moths became abundant, while the lighter coloured moths became rare. He alleged that pollution made the darker moths almost invisible to predatory birds, while the lighter moths became conspicuous. One would expect a larger proportion of the lighter moths to fall prey to these birds. This is an example of selective predation by birds.

In a polluted forest, Kettlewell marked and released 630 male moths: 21.7% were light-coloured and 78.3% were dark-coloured. The released insects were recaptured by assembling to females and at light traps. The proportions of recaptured insects are 13% of the light-coloured moths and 27% of the dark-coloured moths. We select one of the 630 released moths at random.

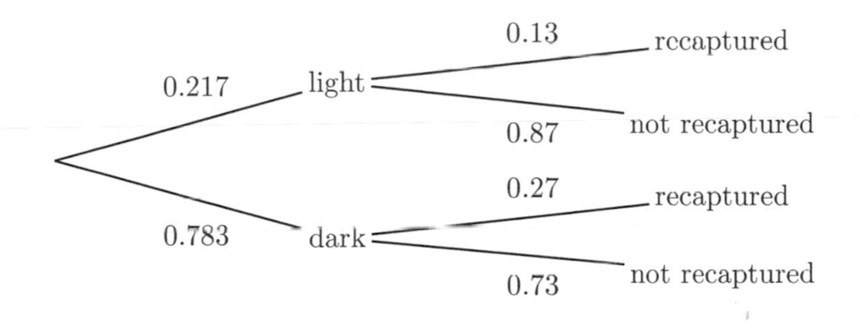

Fig. 4.2 Tree diagram: Peppered moths

Let R be the event that we recapture the moth, L be the event that the moth is light-coloured and D be the event that the moth is dark-coloured.

The probability that we recapture the moth is

$$P(R) = P(R \cap L) + P(R \cap D) = (0.217)(0.13) + (0.783)(0.27) = 23.96\%.$$

The conditional probability that we recapture the moth, given that it is dark-coloured is $P(R|D) = 0.27$. The darker moths have a slightly larger probability of being recaptured.

4.3 Bayes' Rule

Often the sample space S is partitioned into k mutually exclusive events $E_1, E_2, \ldots, E_k$ and we are interested in the probability of another event B. If we know the marginal probabilities $P(E_i)$ and the conditional probabilities $P(B|E_i)$ for $i = 1, \ldots, k$, then we can combine these quantities to obtain the probability that B occurs. This is known as the *total probability rule*:

$$\begin{aligned} P(B) &= P(B \cap E_1) + P(B \cap E_2) + \ldots + P(B \cap E_k) \\ &= P(B|E_1)\,P(E_1) + P(B|E_2)\,P(E_2) + \ldots + P(B|E_k)\,P(E_k). \end{aligned}$$

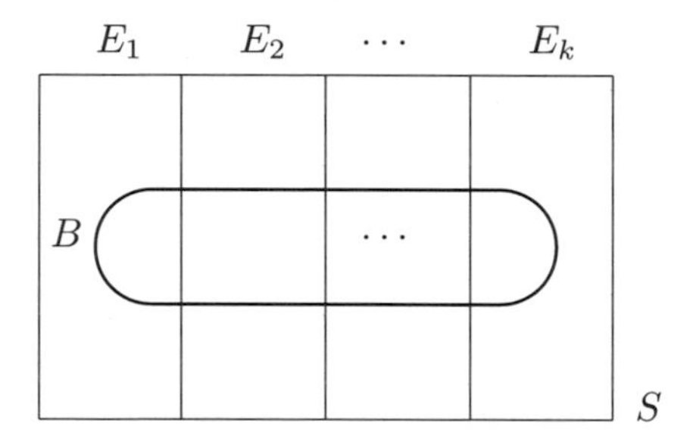

Fig. 4.3 Partitioning the sample space

Example 4.8. Beech trees are abundant in Central Europe. Some beech trees develop "red heartwood" which reduces the timber quality (see [36]). Suppose that in a particular forest, 25% of the beech trees are young, 30% of the trees are moderately aged and 45% of the trees are old. Furthermore, 1% of the young trees develop "red heartwood", while the "red heartwood" rates for the moderately aged and old trees are 25% and 90%, respectively.

The probability that a randomly chosen tree in this forest has formed a "red heartwood" is

$$\begin{aligned} P(R) &= P(R|Y)\,P(Y) + P(R|M)\,P(M) + P(R|O)\,P(O) \\ &= (0.01)(0.25) + (0.25)(0.3) + (0.9)(0.45) = 0.4825. \end{aligned}$$

Here R denotes "red heartwood" and Y, M and O denote "young", "moderately aged" and "old", respectively.

We might want to reverse the conditioning, that is we want to know $P(E_j|B)$ for some j. *Bayes' rule* shows us how to compute this quantity. Bayes' rule is

$$\begin{aligned} P(E_j|B) &= \frac{P(E_j \cap B)}{P(B)} \quad \text{(by definition)} \\ &= \frac{P(B|E_j)\,P(E_j)}{P(B)} \quad \text{(by the multiplication rule)} \\ &= \frac{P(B|E_j)\,P(E_j)}{P(B|E_1)\,P(E_1) + \ldots + P(B|E_k)\,P(E_k)}. \end{aligned}$$

Example 4.8 (Continued). After cutting a tree, we realize that the tree has formed "red heartwood". What is the probability that the tree is old? Using Bayes' rule, we compute

$$P(O|R) = \frac{P(R|O)\,P(O)}{P(R)} = \frac{(0.9)(0.45)}{0.4825} = 0.8394.$$

In the next example, we see that the total probability rule and Bayes' rule can be used to combine information from different studies.

In practice, the computation of the positive (negative) predictive value is a two step process. First, from a study population we can estimate the sensitivity and the specificity of the diagnostic test. However, for many studies the prevalence of the disease for the study population is not the same as the prevalence of the disease for the target population. So the second step is to estimate the prevalence of the disease in the target population with another study.

Example 4.9. [Diagnostic Tests] Suppose that we have 50 subjects with the disease and 50 subjects without the disease. We give the diagnostic test to all the subjects. Among the subjects with the disease, 48 obtained a positive test result. There were only 4 positive results among the subjects without the disease. A summary of the data is found in Table 4.4. A person is selected at random among the 100 subjects. We denote U_+ the event that the person has the disease, U_- the event that the person does not have the disease, T_+ the event of a positive result and T_- the event of a negative result. The sensitivity $P(T_+|U_+) = 48/50 = 96\%$ and the specificity $P(T_-|U_-) = 46/50 = 92\%$ of the test for the study population can be used as estimates of the same metrics for the target population.

Table 4.4 Results for a diagnostic test

	Diseased	Non-diseased
Test +	48	4
Test −	2	46
Total	50	50

Since the subjects were chosen randomly within their respective subpopulation (with and without disease), we should not use the study population to estimate the probability that a subject has the disease. Another study is needed. Suppose that 500 subjects from the target population are randomly chosen and that 45 have the disease. The probability that a subject has the disease is $P(U_+) = 45/500 = 0.09$.

Using Bayes' rule, the positive predictive value for this test is

$$\begin{aligned}\mathsf{PPV} = P(U_+|T_+) &= \frac{P(T_+|U_+)P(U_+)}{P(T_+|U_+)P(U_+) + P(T_+|U_-)P(U_-)} \\ &= \frac{(0.96)(0.09)}{(0.96)(0.09) + (1-0.92)(1-0.09)} = 0.5427.\end{aligned}$$

Example 4.10. [Diagnostic Tests and Rare Diseases] We consider data from Table 4.3. The sensitivity is $P(T_+|U_+) = 0.095/(0.095+0.005) = 0.95$ and the specificity is $P(T_-|U_-) = 0.882/(0.882+0.018) = 0.98$. Consider a population with a prevalence of the disease of only 0.5%. The positive and the negative predictive values are

$$\begin{aligned}\mathsf{PPV} = P(U_+|T_+) &= \frac{P(T_+|U_+)P(U_+)}{P(T_+|U_+)P(U_+) + P(T_+|U_-)P(U_-)} \\ &= \frac{(0.95)(0.005)}{(0.95)(0.005) + (1-0.98)(1-0.005)} = 0.1927,\end{aligned}$$

and respectively we get

$$\begin{aligned}\mathsf{NPV} = P(U_-|T_-) &= \frac{P(T_-|U_-)P(U_-)}{P(T_-|U_+)P(U_+) + P(T_-|U_-)P(U_-)} \\ &= \frac{(0.98)(1-0.005)}{(1-0.95)(0.005) + (0.98)(1-0.005)} = 0.9997.\end{aligned}$$

Despite the fact that the test has high sensitivity and specificity, because the disease is rare the positive predictive value of the test is small. In this example there is a big chance of not having the disease even if the test result is positive.

We end this section with an example from genetics.

Example 4.11. Consider a gene with two alleles A and a, that is not linked with sex. We cross two mice with genotypes Aa. A male offspring that resulted from this cross is crossed with a female with genotype Aa. This new pair has an offspring with the dominant trait. What is the probability that the father is heterozygous?

We denote by H, HR, HD the events that the father is heterozygous (i.e. its genotype is Aa), homozygous recessive (i.e. its genotype is aa), and homozygous dominant (i.e. its genotype is AA), respectively. From Example 2.1, we know that $P(H) = 1/2$, $P(HR) = 1/4$ and $P(HD) = 1/4$. We denote by D the event that the father has an offspring with the dominant trait. Note that $P(D|H) = 3/4$, since when we cross $Aa \times Aa$, 3 of the 4 possible offspring genotypes correspond to an offspring with the dominant trait. $P(D|HR) = 1/2$, since when we cross $Aa \times aa$, 1 of the 2 possible offspring genotypes gives rise to an offspring with the dominant trait. Finally, $P(D|HD) = 1$, since when we cross $Aa \times AA$, all offsprings have the dominant trait.

The probability that the offspring has the dominant trait is

$$\begin{aligned}P(D) &= P(D|H)\,P(H) + P(D|HR)\,P(HR) + P(D|HD)\,P(HD) \\ &= \frac{3}{4}\cdot\frac{1}{2} + \frac{1}{2}\cdot\frac{1}{4} + 1\cdot\frac{1}{4} = \frac{3}{4}.\end{aligned}$$

By Bayes' rule, the probability that the father is heterozygous given that he has an offspring with the dominant trait is

$$P(H|D) = \frac{P(D|H)\,P(H)}{P(D)} = \frac{(3/4)(1/2)}{3/4} = \frac{1}{2}.$$

4.4 Problems

Problem 4.1. One of the objectives of the study [58] was to estimate the probability of developing lung cancer by the smoking status, based on the incidence rates of lung cancer in the Canadian population between 1987 and 1989. It was found that 17.2% of the male smokers and 11.6% of the female smokers will eventually develop lung cancer. In the non-smoker category, 1.3% of the males and 1.4% of the females will develop lung cancer. Knowing that 52.2% of the male population are smokers, and 28.4% of the female population are smokers, find the probability of developing lung cancer for males and females, respectively.

Problem 4.2. The nuchal translucency test is a special ultrasound scan which is widely used as a screening test for Down's syndrome in early pregnancy. The test measures the fluid under the skin at the back of the baby's neck and can be used to determine the risk of having a baby with Down's syndrome. The following table gives the test results for a sample of 1,000 pregnant women, with the age between 35 and 40:

	Down syndrome baby	Normal baby	Total
Test +	3	50	53
Test -	2	945	947
Total	5	995	1,000

Calculate:
(a) the false positive rate and false negative rate of the test;
(b) the sensitivity and specificity of the test;
(c) the positive predictive value and negative predictive value of the test.

Problem 4.3. A screening test which measures the level of a prostate specific antigen (PSA) is a commonly used tool for the detection of prostate cancer. Men with PSA levels greater than 10 (ng/ml) have a chance of 67% of prostate cancer, whereas men whose PSA levels are between 4 and 10 have a 25% chance of having prostate cancer. For those whose PSA levels are below 4, the risk of developing prostate cancer is only 5%. Suppose that 15% of men have PSA levels greater than 10, 10% of men have PSA levels between 4 and 10, and 75% of men have PSA levels lower than 4.
(a) What is the probability that a randomly chosen man will develop prostate cancer?
(b) What is the probability that a randomly chosen man has a PSA level

greater than 10, given that he has prostate cancer?

Problem 4.4. A simple urine test was developed for a particular disease. A study involved 200 patients with the disease and 100 patients without the disease. Among the patients with the disease 197 had a positive result, while there were only 8 positive results among the subjects without the disease.
(a) Calculate the false positive rate and false negative rate of the test.
(b) Calculate the sensitivity and specificity of the test.
(c) Assuming that the prevalence of this disease is 15%, compute the positive predictive value and negative predictive value of the test.
(d) Assuming that the prevalence of this disease is 1%, compute the positive predictive value and negative predictive value of the test.

Problem 4.5. Sickle cell anemia is a genetic blood disorder. Two alleles are important for the inheritance of sickle cell anemia: the sickle allele (S) and the normal adult haemoglobin allele (A) (see [32]). Individuals with two normal A alleles (AA) have normal hemoglobin. Those with two mutant S alleles (SS) develop sickle cell anemia. Those who are heterozygous for the sickle cell allele (AS) produce both normal and abnormal hemoglobin. The heterozygotes are said to have the sickle cell trait. Individuals with the sickle cell trait or anemia are more resistant to malaria. Consider a population in which 20% of the individuals have a sickle cell allele.
(a) Assume that in a certain region, the probability of dying of malaria is 15% for individuals that do not have the sickle cell allele, and 2.5% for individuals with a sickle cell allele. What is the probability of dying of malaria in this region?
(b) If an individual from this population dies from malaria, what is the probability that this individual had a sickle cell allele?

Problem 4.6. About 5% of the population has a cardiovascular disease. Suppose that 75% of the individuals with a cardiovascular disease are not aware of their condition. Compute the probability that an individual from this population has a cardiovascular disease but is not aware of it.

Problem 4.7. Tuberculosis is a rare disease in developing countries. However, it is the most common cause of death in HIV-positive adults living in these countries (see [16]). Consider a country in which 0.045% of its adult population has tuberculosis. It is estimated that 8% of all tuberculosis cases in this country are co-infected with HIV. Compute the probability that a randomly selected adult from this country has both tuberculosis and HIV.

Problem 4.8. Refer to Problem 4.7. It is estimated that 0.16% of the adult population in this country without tuberculosis is infected with HIV.
(a) Compute the probability that a randomly selected adult is infected with HIV.
(b) Given that a randomly selected adult is infected with HIV, compute the probability that this adult is co-infected with tuberculosis.

Did you know that? *It was said many times that Columbus did not prove that the Earth is round; that was already known in 1492. What Columbus proved was that "it doesn't matter how wrong you are, as long as you are lucky" (see [6]). The story says that Columbus was a dreamer whose idea was to find a new route to Asia by sailing to the west. The problem was that nobody knew how long such a trip would be, since the exact figure for the Earth circumference was unknown at the time. The usual estimate for the Earth circumference which was circulated in the Middle Ages was 18,000 miles or 28,968.192 km (which was off by 7,000 miles). Based on this estimate, Columbus managed to convince the king of Spain to fund his trip. It was due to Columbus' incredible luck that his ships reached the ground, after a 3,000 mile trip crossing the Atlantic, which almost killed most of his crewmen and damaged his ships severely. Of course, he was convinced that he reached Asia.*

Chapter 5

Independence

In this chapter we introduce the concept of independent events. Often we are interested in the association between events. For example, does the flu shot change the chances of contracting the flu? If not, we say that the event of contracting the flu is independent of receiving the flu vaccine. We begin with the formal definition of independent events and then motivate this definition with a few examples. We end the chapter by generalizing the notion of independent events to a collection of more than two events.

5.1 Statistical Independence

Definition 5.1. The events A and B are (statistically) **independent** if

$$P(A \cap B) = P(A)\,P(B).$$

One can show that if two events A and B are such that $P(A) > 0$ and $P(B) > 0$, then the following statements are equivalent.

(1) $P(A \cap B) = P(A)\,P(B)$;
(2) $P(A|B) = P(A)$;
(3) $P(B|A) = P(B)$.

By definition, if the equation from statement (1) holds, then the events A and B are independent. Since we cannot condition on an event if it has a probability of zero, statement (1) is more general. Furthermore, as we will see at the end of the chapter, statement (1) is easier to generalize. Statements (2) and (3) mean that the given event does not contain any information concerning the other event, in the sense that the probability of the event of interest does not change even if the other event has occurred. This leads us to a more appealing interpretation of independence. So, if the probability of contracting the flu remains unchanged even if someone receives the flu shot, then we say that the events of getting the flu shot and contracting the flu are independent.

Example 5.1. Consider the foul-hooking Example 4.1. Are the events $F =$"foul-hooking" and $J =$"use of jig" independent? Using the data and the relative frequency approach, we found that: $P(F) = 24\%$ and $P(F|J) = 36.4\%$. Since $P(F) \neq P(F|J)$, the events F and J are not independent. It appears that the use of the jig will increase the chances of foul-hooking a fish.

Note that we do not actually know the true probabilities. Estimation of probabilities (that is population proportions) is discussed in Section 9.2. In Section 9.4, we discuss ways to measure the error of this estimation in a probabilistic sense. In Chapter 14, we introduce a test for independence. Using this test, we will be able to assess the strength of our evidence against independence.

Example 5.2. [Sampling Without Remplacement] According to the Ontario Ministry of the Environment, approximately three million Ontarians depend on wells for their supply of safe drinking water. Consider a small rural community of fifteen households, in which five households have high sodium content in their wells. Select two of these households at random without replacement. Let A_i be the event that the ith selected household has a well with high sodium content, for $i = 1, 2$.

We verify that the events A_1 and A_2 are not independent. The probability that the first well has a high sodium content is $5/15$. Given that the first well has a high sodium content, the conditional probability that the second well has a high sodium content is $P(A_2|A_1) = 4/14 = 0.2860$. However, the (unconditional) probability that the second well has a high sodium content is

$$\begin{aligned} P(A_2) &= P(A_2 \cap A_1) + P(A_2 \cap A_1') \\ &= P(A_2|A_1)P(A_1) + P(A_2|A_1')P(A_1') \\ &= \frac{4}{14} \cdot \frac{5}{15} + \frac{5}{14} \cdot \frac{10}{15} = \frac{1}{3} = 0.3333. \end{aligned}$$

Since $P(A_2) \neq P(A_2|A_1)$, the events A_1 and A_2 are not independent.

Example 5.3. [Sampling Without Remplacement from a Large Population] Refer to Example 5.2. We consider now a larger community of 300 households. We assume that the proportion of households with a high sodium content in their wells is the same as in Example 5.2. If the first selected well has a high sodium content, then the probability that the second well has a high sodium content is $P(A_2|A_1) = 99/299 = 0.3311$. The (unconditional) probability that the second well has a high sodium content is

$$\begin{aligned} P(A_2) &= P(A_2 \cap A_1) + P(A_2 \cap A_1') \\ &= P(A_2|A_1)P(A_1) + P(A_2|A_1')P(A_1') \\ &= \frac{99}{299} \cdot \frac{100}{300} + \frac{100}{299} \cdot \frac{200}{300} = \frac{1}{3} = 0.3333. \end{aligned}$$

Notice that the difference between the conditional and unconditional probabilities is smaller for this larger population. Consider the same question with 3000 households. Then, $P(A_2|A_1) = 999/2999 = 0.3331$ and $P(A_2) = 1/3 = 0.3333$. The statistical dependence between the two trials becomes negligible as the size of the population becomes larger.

When sampling from a large population the statistical dependence between the trials is often negligible. In this case, it is reasonable to consider the trials as independent. The independence of the trials is considered as an underlying assumption of the probability model.

Example 5.4. It is estimated that 46% of Canadians have type O blood and that 15% of Canadians are Rh Negative. Suppose that these are independent events. The proportion of the Canadian population who has Rh Negative blood of type O is

$$P(O-) = P(O)P(\text{Rh}-) = (0.46)(0.15) = 0.069 = 6.9\%.$$

Example 5.5. [Linked Genes and Independent Assortment] We are interested in two different genes, say A and B, and we cross two organisms each with the genotype $AaBb$. Mendel's Law of Independent Assortment states that the alleles of different genes assort independently of each other during gamete formation. This is actually only true for genes that are not linked to each other.

Assuming that the two genes are not linked, compute the probability that an offspring has the genotype $aabb$. When considering only one gene, the cross of two heterozygote parents results in an offspring with a recessive phenotype with a probability of 0.25. By independence $P(\{aabb\}) = P(\{aa\})P(\{bb\}) = (0.25)^2 = 6.25\%$.

In 1913, Alfred Sturtevant, an undergraduate student who worked with Thomas Hunt Morgan, crossed drosophila with genotype $RrWw$, where R = red eyes (r = vermilion eyes) and W = long wings (w = rudimentary wings) (see [54]). He observed that 4 out of 458 (that is 0.09%) offspring have rudimentary wings and vermilion eyes. It appears that wing length and eye colour are linked, since the data is not consistent with the calculations from our model assuming independent assortment.

We now extend the notion of independence to a collection of two or more events.

Definition 5.2. The events $A_1, A_2, \ldots, A_n$ are (mutually) **independent** if for any sub-collection of events $A_{i_1}, A_{i_2}, \ldots, A_{i_k}$, we have

$$P(A_{i_1} \cap A_{i_2} \cap \cdots \cap A_{i_k}) = P(A_{i_1})P(A_{i_2}) \cdots P(A_{i_k}).$$

Fundamental understanding of the random process under study combined with a good judgement enables us to determine when it is sensible to assume that events are independent. If we can assume that certain events are independent, then we can easily compute the probability that all events occur simultaneously, by multiplying the probabilities of the individual events.

The following property is useful in applications. Let $A_1, A_2, \ldots, A_n$ be independent events. We construct a new collection of events as follows. Let B_i be either A_i or A_i', for $i = 1, \ldots, n$. In other words, we keep an event, or we replace it with its complement. Then, $B_1, B_2, \ldots, B_n$ are independent events.

In particular, if A and B are independent, then

- A and B' are independent;
- A' and B are independent;
- A' and B' are independent.

Example 5.6. A particular medical procedure has an 85% success rate. Four patients undergo the procedure. What is the probability that the operation is successful for all four? What is the probability that it is successful for at least one of the patients? What is the probability that only the first operation is successful?

We assume that the results of these operations are mutually independent. Let A_i be the event that the ith operation is successful, for $i = 1, 2, 3, 4$. By independence, the probability that all the operations are successful is $P(A_1 \cap \cdots \cap A_4) = P(A_1) \cdots P(A_4) = (0.85)^4 = 0.5220$. The probability that at least one of the operations is successful is

$$\begin{aligned} P(A_1 \cup \cdots \cup A_4) &= 1 - P[(A_1 \cup \cdots \cup A_4)'] = 1 - P(A_1' \cap \cdots \cap A_4') \\ &= 1 - P(A_1') \cdots P(A_4') = 1 - (1 - 0.85)^4 = 0.9995. \end{aligned}$$

The probability that only the first operation is successful is $P(A_1 \cap A_2' \cap A_3' \cap A_4') = (0.85)(0.15)^3 = 0.0029$.

5.2 Problems

Problem 5.1. It is known that in Canada, the blood types have the following distribution: 46% O, 42% A, 9% B, 3% AB. A randomly chosen Canadian receives a blood transfusion. Knowing that O is a universal donor, A can donate only to A and AB, B can donate only to B and AB, and AB can donate only to AB, what is the probability that the transfusion is not successful?

Problem 5.2. Whooping cranes are the tallest North American birds. Due to the loss of their habitat, they are on the list of endangered species since 1967. The birds nest and lay eggs in the Wood Buffalo National Park (Northern Alberta, Canada) and then migrate 2,500 miles south to spend the winter in Texas. Recent statistics released by the Canadian Wildlife Services show that the flock population has reached 266 in the spring of 2008, but 57 have died by the following spring (see [31]). Five cranes are tagged, and then released in the wilderness. Assuming that their survival is independent of each other, what is the probability that all five birds will be alive by the next spring? What is the probability that none of them will survive by the next spring?

Problem 5.3. Depression is a mood disorder which is usually associated with significant mental health problems. In Canada, it is estimated that in the population of ages 15 to 64, 16% of women and 8% of men suffer from depression. According to census data released by Statistics Canada in October 2009, the ratio between the male and female populations for the Canadian adults aged 15 to 64 is 0.83.
(a) What percentage of the Canadian population aged 15 to 64 consists of females?
(b) What is the probability that a randomly chosen person of age 15 to 64 suffers from depression?

(c) Is depression independent of gender?
(d) What is the probability that a randomly chosen person is a female, given that the person suffers from depression?

Problem 5.4. Consider two events A and B such that $P(A) > 0$ and $P(B) > 0$. Show that the following two statements are equivalent:

(a) $P(A \cap B) = P(A)P(B)$;
(b) $P(A|B) = P(A)$.

Problem 5.5. To compare two varieties of barley (b_1 and b_2), an experiment is conducted on five equally sized plots. For each plot, we flip a coin to determine which variety to use. We use variety b_1 if the coin comes up heads, and variety b_2 if the coin comes up tails. Suppose that the probability that the coin lands on heads is 0.6. Compute the probability that
(a) b_1 is used only in the first plot;
(b) b_1 is used in all five plots;
(c) the same variety of barley is used in all five plots.

Problem 5.6. Consider a diagnostic test for a certain type of cancer, which has a false positive rate of 5% and a false negative rate of 4%. Assume that 5% of the population has this type of cancer.
(a) If a randomly selected person has a positive test result, what is the probability that the person has this type of cancer?
(b) The test is administered twice on the same patient. Assume that the test results are independent of each other, conditionally on the patient's disease status. Given that both test results are positive, what is the probability that the patient has this type of cancer?
(c) The test is administered four times on the same patient. Assume that the test results are independent of each other, conditionally on the patient's disease status. Given that at least one of the four test results is positive, what is the probability that the patient has this type of cancer?

Did you know that? *Thomas Hunt Morgan was awarded the Nobel Prize in Physiology/Medicine in 1933. The work for which the prize was awarded was completed over a 17-year period at Columbia University, commencing in 1910 with his discovery of the white-eyed mutation in the fruit fly, Drosophila. He showed that genes are linked in a series on chromosomes and are responsible for identifiable, hereditary traits.*

Chapter 6

Discrete Random Variables

A random variable is a measurement whose value is determined by chance. A random variable which can take only a finite (or infinite, but countable) number of values is called *discrete*. Examples of discrete random variables are: the sex of a newborn child, the blood type of an individual, the number of genes A in an offspring of two heterozygous individuals Aa, etc. A random variable whose set of possible values is uncountable is called *continuous*. Examples of continuous random variables are: the weight (or height) of an individual, the blood pressure (or temperature) of a patient, the weight gain of a woman during pregnancy, etc. We denote random variables with capital letters X, Y, Z, etc. and their values with small letters x, y, z, etc.

In the present chapter we study the discrete random variables. Continuous random variables will be studied in Chapter 7.

6.1 Definition

A discrete random variable is characterized by the set of its possible values, and the associated probabilities. For example, if X is the sex of a newborn child, then X can take only two values (male and female), and the associated probabilities are 0.5 and 0.5. These probabilities are represented in a table format, as follows:

x	male	female
$P(X = x)$	0.5	0.5

The function which gives the probabilities associated to all the possible values of X is called *the probability mass function*:

$$f(x) = P(X = x).$$

Note that if x is an impossible value for X, then $f(x) = 0$. Moreover, since $f(x)$ are probabilities, we have:

$$0 \leq f(x) \leq 1 \quad \text{and} \quad \sum_x f(x) = 1,$$

where the sum is taken over all the possible values x of X. The table (or graph) summarizing the values of $f(x)$ is called the *distribution* of X.

The *cumulative distribution function* $F(x)$ gives the probability that X takes values smaller than or equal to x:

$$F(x) = P(X \leq x) = \sum_{y \leq x} f(y).$$

Example 6.1. The number of days with sunshine in Ottawa, in the month of January is a random variable X which takes the values $0, 1, 2, 3, \ldots, 30, 31$. Based on the data collected in the past 50 years, the values smaller than 12 or larger than 20 have probability 0. The values between 12 and 20 have non-zero probabilities given by the following table:

x	12	13	14	15	16	17	18	19	20
$f(x)$	0.07	0.03	0.13	0.15	0.2	0.04	0.01	0.07	0.3

The function $f(x)$ is represented graphically in Figure 6.1.

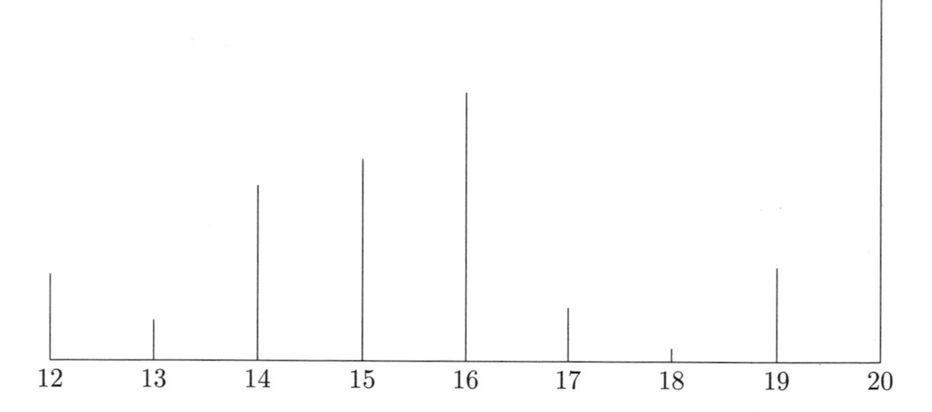

Fig. 6.1 The probability mass function $f(x)$ of the number of days with sunshine

For values x which are not in the table, $f(x) = 0$. For instance, $f(13.5) = P(X = 13.5) = 0$, since 13.5 is an impossible value for X.

The following table gives the cumulative distribution function $F(x)$ of X:

x	12	13	14	15	16	17	18	19	20
$F(x)$	0.07	0.1	0.23	0.38	0.58	0.62	0.63	0.7	1.00

For values x which are not in the table, $F(x)$ is not necessarily 0. For instance,

$$F(13.5) = P(X \leq 13.5) = P(X \leq 13) = F(13) = 0.1.$$

The probability that this year in January, there will be at least 17 days with sunshine in Ottawa, is:

$$\begin{aligned} P(X \geq 17) &= P(X = 17) + P(X = 18) + P(X = 19) + P(X = 20) \\ &= 0.04 + 0.01 + 0.07 + 0.3 = 0.42. \end{aligned}$$

Alternatively, this probability can be calculated as:

$$P(X \geq 17) = 1 - P(X \leq 16) = 1 - F(16) = 1 - 0.58 = 0.42.$$

The probability that there will be at most 14 days with sunshine in Ottawa in January, is

$$\begin{aligned} P(X \leq 14) = F(14) &= P(X = 12) + P(X = 13) + P(X = 14) \\ &= 0.07 + 0.03 + 0.13 = 0.23. \end{aligned}$$

The function $F(x)$ is represented graphically in Figure 6.1.

The average value of a random variable X is called the *expectation* (or *expected value*, or *mean*) of X, and is denoted by $\mu = E(X)$. Whereas the exact value taken by a discrete random variable X is unknown (since it is random), its expectation is non-random and can be calculated by the following formula:

$$\mu = E(X) = \sum_x x f(x).$$

The average squared difference between X and $E(X)$ is called the *variance* of X, and is denoted by $\sigma^2 = \text{Var}(X)$. In the case of a discrete random variable, the variance is calculated by the formula:

$$\sigma^2 = \text{Var}(X) = \sum_x (x - \mu)^2 f(x).$$

Alternatively, the variance can be calculated by the formula:

$$\sigma^2 = \text{Var}(X) = E(X^2) - \mu^2 = \sum_x x^2 f(x) - \mu^2,$$

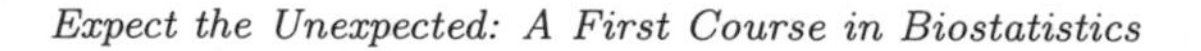

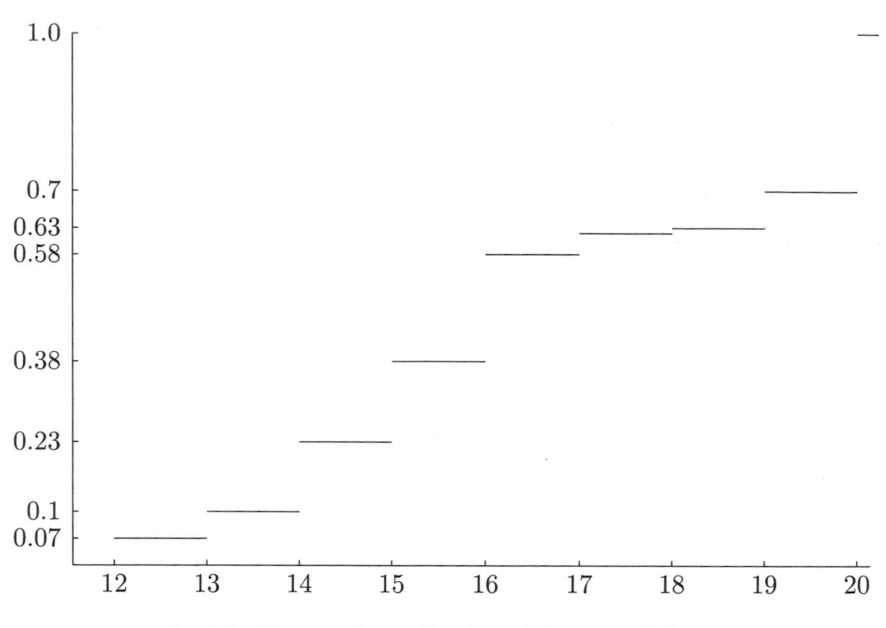

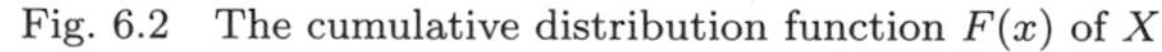
Fig. 6.2 The cumulative distribution function $F(x)$ of X

where $E(X^2)$ is the expectation of the variable X^2.

The square root σ of the variance is called the *standard deviation* of X:

$$\sigma = \sqrt{\text{Var}(X)}.$$

The standard deviation σ of a random variable X is a measure of the amount of variability in the values of X around the average value $\mu = E(X)$. A small value of σ indicates that on the average, X is close to $E(X)$.

Example 6.1 (Continued). The expected (or average) number of days with sunshine in Ottawa in January is:

$$\begin{aligned}\mu = E(X) &= 12(0.07) + 13(0.03) + 14(0.13) + 15(0.15) + 16(0.2)\\ &\quad + 17(0.04) + 18(0.01) + 19(0.07) + 20(0.3)\\ &= 16.69.\end{aligned}$$

The variance of X is:

$$\begin{aligned}\sigma^2 = \text{Var}(X) &= 12^2(0.07) + 13^2(0.03) + 14^2(0.13) + 15^2(0.15) + 16^2(0.2)\\ &\quad + 17^2(0.04) + 18^2(0.01) + 19^2(0.07) + 20^2(0.3) - (16.69)^2\\ &= 285.65 - 278.56\\ &= 7.0939.\end{aligned}$$

The standard deviation of X is: $\sigma = \sqrt{7.0939} = 2.663$.

6.2 Binomial Distribution

Consider 4 tosses of a fair coin, and let X be the number of heads. X is a discrete random variable whose possible values are: $0, 1, 2, 3, 4$. But what are the probabilities associated to these values?

The probability that $X = 0$ (no heads) is:

$$P(X = 0) = P(\text{tail})P(\text{tail})P(\text{tail})P(\text{tail}) = (0.5)^4 = 0.0625.$$

The event $X = 1$ (one head) is the union of 4 disjoint events:
$A_1 = \{\text{head}, \text{tail}, \text{tail}, \text{tail}\}$, $A_2 = \{\text{tail}, \text{head}, \text{tail}, \text{tail}\}$,
$A_3 = \{\text{tail}, \text{tail}, \text{head}, \text{tail}\}$, $A_4 = \{\text{tail}, \text{tail}, \text{tail}, \text{head}\}$.

Note that

$$P(A_1) = P(\text{head})P(\text{tail})P(\text{tail})P(\text{tail}) = (0.5)(0.5)^3 = 0.0625.$$

A similar calculation shows that $P(A_2) = P(A_3) = P(A_4) = 0.0625$. Hence

$$P(X = 1) = 4(0.0625) = 0.25.$$

The event $X = 2$ (two heads) is the union of 6 disjoint events, 6 corresponding to $\binom{4}{2}$, the number of ways of choosing the 2 heads among the 4 possible trials (see Section 2.2). The 6 events are:
$B_1 = \{\text{head}, \text{head}, \text{tail}, \text{tail}\}$, $B_2 = \{\text{head}, \text{tail}, \text{head}, \text{tail}\}$,
$B_3 = \{\text{head}, \text{tail}, \text{tail}, \text{head}\}$, $B_4 = \{\text{tail}, \text{head}, \text{head}, \text{tail}\}$,
$B_5 = \{\text{tail}, \text{head}, \text{tail}, \text{head}\}$, $B_6 = \{\text{tail}, \text{tail}, \text{head}, \text{head}\}$.

Note that

$$P(B_1) = P(\text{head})P(\text{head})P(\text{tail})P(\text{tail}) = (0.5)^2(0.5)^2 = 0.0625.$$

A similar calculation shows that $P(B_i) = 0.0625$ for any $i = 2, \ldots, 6$. Hence

$$P(X = 2) = 6(0.0625) = 0.375.$$

Arguing in the same way, we infer that:

$$P(X = 3) = \binom{4}{3}(0.5)^3(0.5) = 4(0.0625) = 0.25$$

$$P(X = 4) = (0.5)^4 = 0.0625.$$

Summarizing, we obtain the following table for the probability mass function $f(x)$ of X:

x	0	1	2	3	4
$f(x)$	0.0625	0.25	0.375	0.25	0.0625

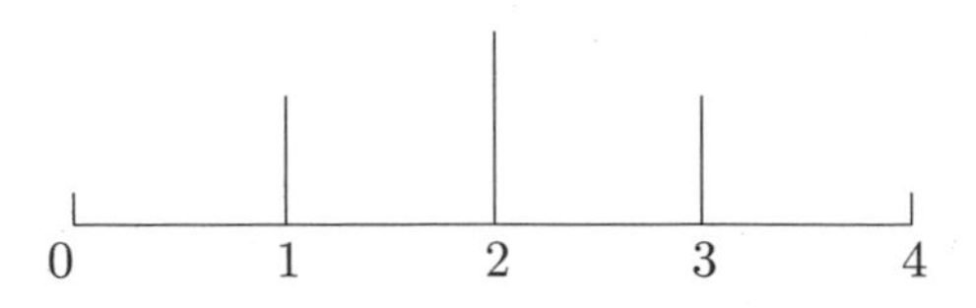

Fig. 6.3 The probability mass function $f(x)$ of the number of heads

The previous example illustrates a more general situation. Consider a random experiment with only two possible results, called "success" and "failure", such that the probability of success is p, and hence, the probability of failure is $1-p$. The experiment is repeated n times, such that the results obtained in the n trials are independent of each other. Let X be the number of successes. Then, X is a discrete random variable, which takes the values $0, 1, 2, \ldots, n$ with the following probabilities:

$$P(X = k) = \binom{n}{k} p^k (1-p)^{n-k}, \quad \text{for any} \quad k = 0, 1, 2, \ldots, n.$$

We say that X has a *binomial distribution* with n trials and probability p of success. One can show that

$$E(X) = np \quad \text{and} \quad \mathrm{Var}(X) = np(1-p).$$

Example 6.2. A new treatment for kidney cancer has a 60% chance of giving good results. A group of 5 patients are given this treatment. Let X be the number of patients for whom the treatment gives good results. X is a discrete random variable with possible values $0, 1, 2, 3, 4, 5$. Since each treatment may have only two results, and the results of the 5 treatments are independent of each other, X has a binomial distribution with $n = 5$ trials and probability $p = 0.6$ of success. The probabilities associated to the values $k = 0, 1, 2, 3, 4, 5$ are calculated by the following formula:

$$P(X = k) = \binom{5}{k} (0.6)^k (0.4)^{5-k}.$$

More precisely,

$$P(X=0) = \binom{5}{0}(0.6)^0(0.4)^{5-0} = (0.4)^5 = 0.01024$$

$$P(X=1) = \binom{5}{1}(0.6)^1(0.4)^{5-1} = 5(0.6)(0.4)^4 = 0.0768$$

$$P(X=2) = \binom{5}{2}(0.6)^2(0.4)^{5-2} = 10(0.6)^2(0.4)^3 = 0.2304$$

$$P(X=3) = \binom{5}{3}(0.6)^3(0.4)^{5-3} = 10(0.6)^3(0.4)^2 = 0.3456$$

$$P(X=4) = \binom{5}{4}(0.6)^4(0.4)^{5-4} = 5(0.6)^4(0.4) = 0.2592$$

$$P(X=5) = \binom{5}{5}(0.6)^5(0.4)^{5-5} = (0.6)^5 = 0.07776.$$

These probabilities are summarized by the table below:

x	0	1	2	3	4	5
$f(x)$	0.01024	0.0768	0.2304	0.3456	0.2592	0.07776

Below is the graph of the probability mass function:

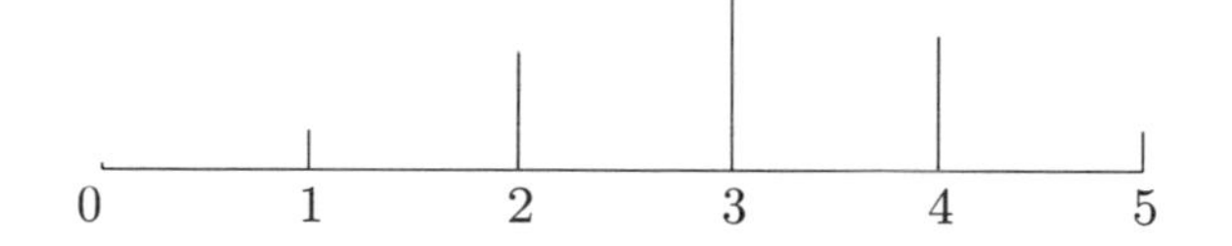

Fig. 6.4 The probability mass function $f(x)$ of the number of patients

The probability that there are at least 3 patients in the group for which the treatment will give good results is:

$$\begin{aligned} P(X \geq 3) &= P(X=3) + P(X=4) + P(X=5) \\ &= 0.3456 + 0.2592 + 0.07776 = 0.6826. \end{aligned}$$

The expectation and variance of X are:

$$E(X) = 5(0.6) = 3 \quad \text{and} \quad \text{Var}(X) = 5(0.6)(0.4) = 1.2.$$

Example 6.3. 0.03% of the population is allergic to a compound found in a flu vaccine. A group of 7 persons are given this vaccine. Let X be the number of people who have an adverse reaction to the vaccine (among the

7 persons). X has a binomial distribution with $n = 7$ trials and probability $p = 0.0003$ of success. The associated probabilities are given by the following formula:

$$P(X = k) = \binom{7}{k} (0.0003)^k (0.9997)^{7-k}, \quad \text{for any} \quad k = 0, 1, 2, 3, 4, 5, 6, 7.$$

The probability that at least one person in this group has an adverse reaction to the vaccine is:

$$P(X \geq 1) = 1 - P(X = 0) = 1 - (0.9997)^7 = 0.002.$$

6.3 Poisson Distribution

Consider a sequence of events which occur at random moments of time. For instance, these events could be the arrivals of patients at the emergency room of a hospital, the occurrences of earthquakes in a certain region, the telephone calls regarding an ad posted in a newspaper, etc. Suppose that:

- the number of events which occur in disjoint time intervals are independent of each other; and
- the average number of events occurring in any fixed time interval is proportional to the length of the interval, i.e. it is equal to a constant λ times the length of the interval.

In this case, we say that the events occur according to a *Poisson process.* The random variable X which gives the number of events occurring in one unit of time has a *Poisson distribution* with parameter λ. More precisely, X is a discrete random variable which takes the values $0, 1, 2, 3, \ldots$ with the following probabilities:

$$P(X = k) = e^{-\lambda} \frac{\lambda^k}{k!}, \quad \text{for any} \quad k = 0, 1, 2, 3, \ldots$$

Here e denotes Euler's number, i.e. $e = 2.71828\ldots$. It is defined as

$$e = \lim_{n \to \infty} \left(1 + \frac{1}{n}\right)^n.$$

One can show that the expectation and the variance of X are given by:

$$E(X) = \lambda \quad \text{and} \quad \text{Var}(X) = \lambda.$$

Let Y be the number of events occurring in s units of time. Then Y has a Poisson distribution with parameter λs, i.e. Y is a discrete random variable which takes the values $0, 1, 2, 3, \ldots$ with probabilities:

$$P(Y = k) = e^{-\lambda s}\frac{(\lambda s)^k}{k!}, \quad \text{for any} \quad k = 0, 1, 2, 3, \ldots$$

Example 6.4. During the day, patients arrive at the emergency room of a hospital at the average rate of $\lambda = 6$ patients per hour. Suppose that the patients' arrivals occur according to a Poisson process. Let X be the number of patients who arrive between 1 p.m. and 2 p.m. Then X has a Poisson distribution with parameter $\lambda = 6$.

The probability that there are at most 3 patients arriving between 1 p.m. and 2 p.m. is:

$$\begin{aligned} P(X \le 3) &= P(X = 0) + P(X = 1) + P(X = 2) + P(X = 3) \\ &= e^{-6} + e^{-6}\frac{6}{1!} + e^{-6}\frac{6^2}{2!} + e^{-6}\frac{6^3}{3!} \\ &= 0.002479 + 0.014873 + 0.044618 + 0.089235 = 0.1512. \end{aligned}$$

The registration process of one patient takes 5 minutes. If during this time a new patient arrives, a line-up starts to build up. We want to calculate the probability that this happens. Let Y be the number of patients arriving in 5 minutes. Note that 5 minutes represent $s = 1/12$ of an hour. (The hour is the unit of time in this example.) Then, Y has a Poisson distribution with parameter

$$\lambda s = 6 \cdot \frac{1}{12} = 0.5.$$

The probability that there are at least 2 patients arriving in 5 minutes (and hence a line-up starts to build up), is:

$$\begin{aligned} P(Y \ge 2) &= 1 - P(Y \le 1) = 1 - P(Y = 0) - P(Y = 1) \\ &= 1 - e^{-0.5} - e^{-0.5}\frac{0.5}{1!} \\ &= 1 - 0.60653 - 0.30326 = 1 - 0.9098 = 0.0902. \end{aligned}$$

In other words, even if on average there is only "half a patient" arriving in 5 minutes, there is a chance of 9.02% that there is a line-up.

6.4 Problems

Problem 6.1. A group of primatologists studied the behavior of chimpanzees in the Congolese rain forest. Using a sophisticated set of tools, the chimps managed after several trials to reach a honey hive hidden deep in a hard-to-access crevice. Let X be the number of trials needed by a randomly chosen chimp to reach the honey hive. According to the primatologists' data, X is a random variable with the following distribution:

X	2	3	4	5	6	7
$P(X = x)$	0.05	0.25	0.3	0.2	0.1	0.1

(a) What is the probability that a chimp will reach the honey hive after at least 5 trials?
(b) What is the probability that a chimp will reach the honey hive before at most 3 trials?
(c) What is the expected number of trials needed by a chip to reach the honey hive?
(d) What is the variance of X?

Problem 6.2. Epilepsy is a chronic neurological disorder characterized by recurrent seizures. A large proportion of people with epilepsy do not have seizure control even with the best available medications. The following table gives the distribution of the number of seizures per year for a sample of 500 epilepsy patients who are using the same medication:

Number of seizures per year	Frequency (Number of patients)
0	325
1	108
2	35
3	21
4	11
Total	500

Let X be the number of seizures per year of a randomly chosen patient in this group.
(a) Find the probability mass function of X.
(b) Calculate $P(X \geq 3)$.
(c) Calculate $E(X)$.

Problem 6.3. In humans, the eye color is determined by a gene whose allele for brown eyes is dominant over the allele for blue eyes. A man and a woman have brown eyes, but they are heterozygous for this gene. They have three children. Calculate the probability that:
(a) all three children have blue eyes;

(b) none of their children have blue eyes;
(c) at least one child has blue eyes.

Problem 6.4. Suppose that the number of fatalities due to bear attacks in North America can be modeled as a Poisson random variable with an average of $\lambda = 2$ deaths per year.
(a) What is the probability that there will be no fatalities due to a bear attack in North America in the following two years?
(b) What is the probability that there will be at most one fatality due to a bear attack in the next three years?

Problem 6.5. Consider a new medication for a particular type of short term pain. The medication was given to 20 patients and 17 reported a significant reduction in their pain. Such pain does subside for about 50% of all patients even without medication. Assuming that the medication has no effect in terms of reducing the pain, compute the probability that at least 17 of 20 patients would report a significant reduction in their pain.

Problem 6.6. Sturgeon is a name used to describe a family of fish. It is one of the oldest fish families in Canada, dating back 200 million years. They have undergone little change over time and are often described as living fossils (see [22]). Typical adult sturgeons are between 2 meters and 6 meters long. Sturgeons are bottom feeders that eat mainly crustaceans and small shells. As they grow larger they may eat other fish and depending on their size, they can even swallow a whole salmon. Assume that 45% of the sturgeons in a particular river are large enough to swallow a whole salmon. If 10 sturgeons are randomly selected from this river, what is the probability that
(a) none is large enough to swallow a whole salmon;
(b) at least one is large enough to swallow a whole salmon;
(c) between 2 and 5, inclusively, are large enough to swallow a whole salmon.

Problem 6.7. Most female black bears have their first mating between the ages of 3 and 5 years old. From a large sample of female black bears, we construct the following distribution for X, the size of a litter.

size of litter	probability
1	0.105
2	0.512
3	0.330
4	0.052
5	0.001

(a) Compute the expected size of a litter.
(b) Compute the probability that a litter is at most 2 cubs.

Problem 6.8. Refer to Problem 6.7. Suppose that we select 10 litters at random. Let Y be the number of litters with at least 2 cubs.
(a) What is the expected value of the random variable Y?
(b) What is the probability that Y is at most 3?
(c) What is the probability that three of the litters have exactly one cub?

Did you know that? *Jane Goodall is a British anthropologist who became known worldwide due to her 50 years of research on chimpanzees. Having no conventional university training, but with a self-taught solid knowledge about animals, the 26-year old Goodall was recruited in 1960 by Louis Leakey (a famous paleo-anthropologist) to help his team in the search for early humans fossils in Eastern Africa. In the years that follow, she began to observe the chimpanzee behavior in Gombe Stream National Park (Tanzania). A pioneer in this field, she patiently developed her own methods of observing both social groups and individual chimpanzees over long periods of time, making breakthrough discoveries about their behavior. One of her major discoveries was the fact that chimps devise and use simple tools, a discovery which has prompted the scientific community to redefine the term "human being". Due to her extensive field work, Jane Goodall received a doctorate from Cambridge University, without having earned an undergraduate degree. In the later years, Jane Goodall has turned her attention to the problem of chimps in captivity, which are used for laboratory testing, due to their resemblance to human beings. One of her famous quotes is: "You cannot share your life with any animal with a well-developed brain and not realize that animals have personalities." More details about Jane Goodall's extraordinary life can be found in* [26].

Chapter 7

Continuous Random Variables

In Chapter 6, we studied discrete random variables, i.e. variables whose range is countable. In this chapter, we consider variables that can take values in an interval of real numbers. Such variables are called *continuous*. Examples of continuous random variables are: the length, the area, the volume, the pressure, the temperature, the mass, and many others. We end the chapter with the normal distribution which plays an important role in statistics.

7.1 Definition

To specify the probabilities associated with the values of a continuous random X, we use its cumulative distribution function, which is defined as $F(x) = P(X \leq x)$, where x is a real number.

For discrete random variables, the cumulative distribution function is a non-decreasing step function (see Figure 6.1). In the case of a discrete random variable X, the probability associated to the values of X are added in steps for calculating $F(x)$. In the case of a continuous random variable, the function F does not have any jumps, and cumulates continuously. This motivates the following definition.

Let X be a random variable with the cumulative distribution function F. The random variable X is *continuous* if F is a continuous function. Its *probability density function* is defined by:

$$f(x) = \begin{cases} F'(x), & \text{if } F'(x) \text{ exists,} \\ 0, & \text{otherwise,} \end{cases}$$

where F' is the derivative function of F. In other words, the function f is the rate at which the probabilities are cumulated. The shape of the graph of the density function f is referred to as the *distribution* of X. The function f has the following properties:

$$f(x) \geq 0 \text{ for all } x, \quad \int_{-\infty}^{\infty} f(x)\,dx = 1.$$

By the Fundamental Theorem of Calculus, we obtain another interpretation of the density:

$$P(a < X \leq b) = P(X \leq b) - P(X \leq a) = F(b) - F(a) = \int_a^b f(x)\,dx.$$

So the probability that X falls in the interval $\{x : a < x \leq b\}$ is the area under the graph of f from $x = a$ to $x = b$. Refer to Figure 7.1 for a graphical example of a cumulative distribution function $F(x)$ of a random variable X that takes values in the interval $[0, 1]$, and the corresponding probability density function $f(x)$.

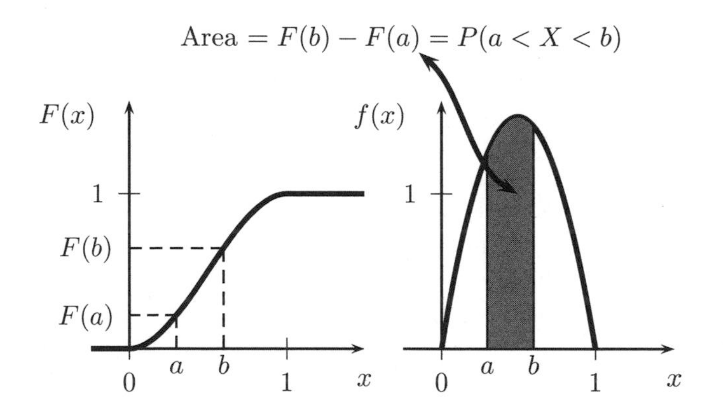

Fig. 7.1 A cumulative distribution function and its associated density

For a continuous random variable X, we must assign a probability of zero to a single value x (which can be considered as an interval of length zero). In other words, $P(X = x) = 0$, for any real number x. The consequence of assigning zero probabilities to single values x is that we can include (or exclude) a value to an interval, and the probability remains the same. Thus,

$$F(x) = P(X \leq x) = P(X < x)$$

and

$$\begin{aligned} F(b) - F(a) &= P(a < X \leq b) = P(a < X < b) \\ &= P(a \leq X \leq b) = P(a \leq X < b). \end{aligned}$$

As in the discrete case, the central tendency of a continuous random variable X is described by its *expectation* μ (also called the *expected value* or *mean*), defined as

$$\mu = E(X) = \int_{-\infty}^{\infty} x\, f(x)\, dx.$$

The mean is a weighted average of the possible values taken by the random variable. The more likely the value, the larger its contribution to the weighted average. Furthermore, the mean is the centre of mass of the distribution.

To describe the dispersion of the random variable, we use the following measure called the *variance*:

$$\sigma^2 = \mathrm{Var}(X) = E[(X - \mu)^2] = \int_{-\infty}^{\infty} (x - \mu)^2\, f(x)\, dx.$$

Alternatively, the variance can be calculated as:

$$\sigma^2 = \mathrm{Var}(X) = E(X^2) - \mu^2 = \int_{-\infty}^{\infty} x^2\, f(x)\, dx - \mu^2,$$

where $E(X^2)$ is the expectation of X^2.

The variance is the expected squared deviation away from the mean. A more dispersed distribution should have a larger variance. Since squared units are difficult to interpret, we compute the square root of the variance. This computation gives the *standard deviation* of X defined as

$$\sigma = \sqrt{\mathrm{Var}(X)}.$$

Figure 7.2 gives the graph of the density functions which correspond to two continuous random variables. The random variable with a mean of 25 has a distribution which is less dispersed. Its values are more concentrated about the mean compared to the other random variable. This random variable has a smaller standard deviation. More precisely, the random variable on the left has a mean of 25 and a standard deviation of 5, while the random variable on the right has a mean of 30 and a standard deviation of 10.

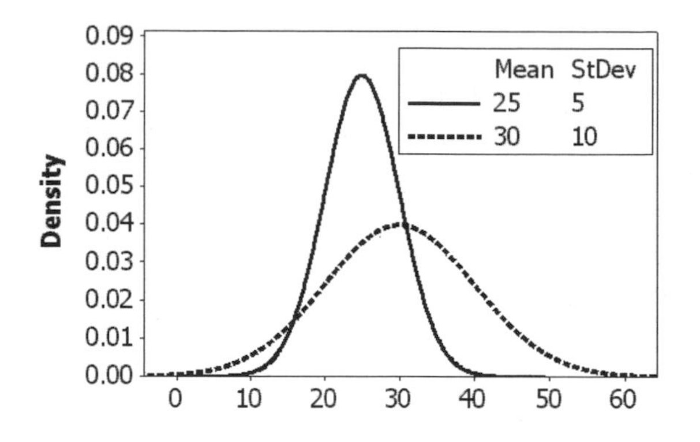

Fig. 7.2 Distributions with different means and standard deviations

7.2 Normal Distribution

In this section, we introduce the normal random distribution, which is often used as an approximation for the distribution of a measurement arising from a random experiment. This is often (but not always) a reasonable assumption. The crucial role played by the normal distribution for the statistical inference will become clear in Section 9.2.

We say that a continuous random variable X has a *normal distribution* with parameters μ and σ if its probability density function is given by:

$$f(x) = \frac{1}{\sigma\sqrt{2\pi}}\, e^{-(x-\mu)^2/(2\sigma^2)}, \quad -\infty < x < \infty,$$

where $-\infty < \mu < \infty$ and $\sigma > 0$.

It can be shown that, if X is a normal random variable with parameters μ and σ, then

$$E(X) = \mu \quad \text{and} \quad \mathrm{Var}(X) = \sigma^2.$$

We use the notation $X \sim N(\mu, \sigma^2)$ when X has a normal distribution with mean μ and variance σ^2.

Properties of a Normal Density:

- The graph of the density of a normal random variable is a symmetric, bell-shaped curve centered about its mean μ (see Figure 7.3).
- Using the method of substitution with $z = (x-\mu)/\sigma$, we get

$$\int_{\mu-k\sigma}^{\mu+k\sigma} \frac{1}{\sigma\sqrt{2\pi}} e^{-\frac{1}{2}\left(\frac{x-\mu}{\sigma}\right)^2} dx = \int_{-k}^{k} \frac{1}{\sqrt{2\pi}}\, e^{-z^2/2}\, dz. \tag{7.1}$$

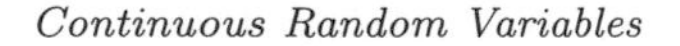

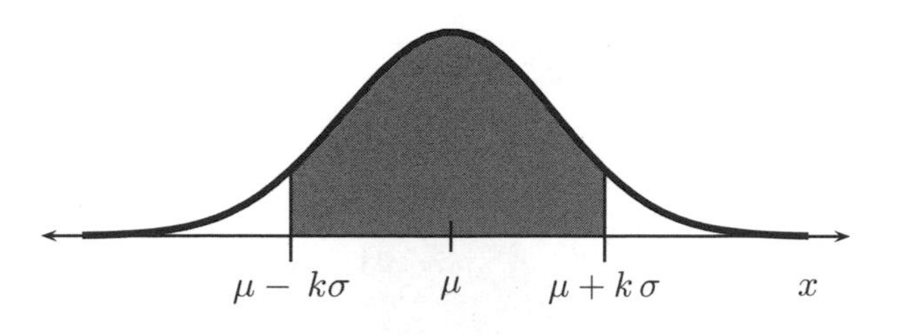

Fig. 7.3 A normal density

Regardless of the value of μ and σ, the probability of being within k standard deviations from the mean is always the same (see Figure 7.3 for a graphical representation).

- The probability that X is within 1 standard deviation from the mean is about 68%. The probability that X is within 2 standard deviations from the mean is about 95%. The probability that X is within 3 standard deviations from the mean is about 99.7%.
- A normal random variable Z with mean 0 and variance 1 is called *standard normal*. Its density is given by:

$$f(z) = \frac{1}{\sqrt{2\,\pi}}\, e^{-z^2/2}, \quad -\infty < z < \infty.$$

Its cumulative distribution function is denoted by Φ, i.e.

$$\Phi(z) = P(Z \leq z), \quad \text{where } Z \sim N(0,1).$$

The values of the cumulative distribution function of the standard normal distribution are found in Tables 17.2 and 17.3.

Example 7.1. Consider a standard normal random variable Z. We will compute the probability that Z falls between -1.25 and 0.5. Refer to Figure 7.4 for a graphical representation of the problem.

When using Tables 17.2 and 17.3, we round the z-values to two decimal places. To use these tables, first start by considering the value at one decimal place to determine the appropriate row, and then the value of the second decimal to determine the column. From Table 17.2, we get $\Phi(-1.25) = 0.1056$. From Table 17.3, we get $\Phi(0.5) = 0.6915$. Therefore,

$$P(-1.25 < Z < 0.5) = \Phi(0.5) - \Phi(-1.25) = 0.6915 - 0.1056 = 0.5859.$$

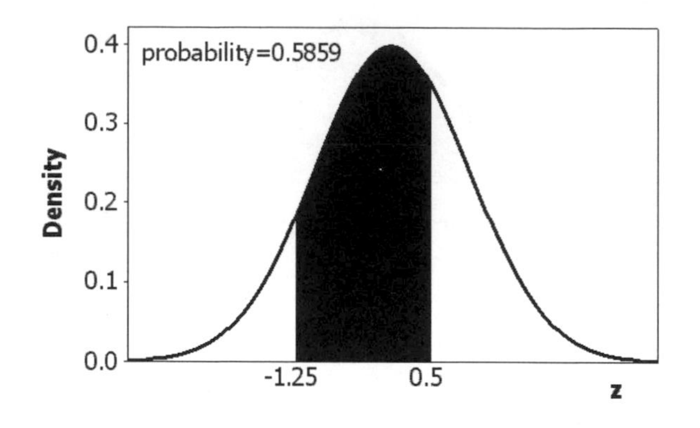

Fig. 7.4 Area under the standard normal density

Theorem 7.1 (Standardization Theorem). *Consider a random variable X with mean μ and standard deviation σ. The standardization of X is*

$$Z = \frac{X - \mu}{\sigma}.$$

The standardized random variable Z has a mean of zero and a variance equal to one. Furthermore, if X is normally distributed, then Z is a standard normal random variable. As a consequence

$$P(X \leq a) = P\left(Z \leq \frac{a - \mu}{\sigma}\right) = \Phi\left(\frac{a - \mu}{\sigma}\right).$$

Example 7.2. Suppose that the length of fish from a particular cohort is normally distributed with a mean of 40 cm and a standard deviation of 3 cm.

(a) What percentage of fish from this cohort are longer than 45 cm?
(b) What is the probability that a randomly selected fish from this cohort is between 37 cm and 43 cm in length?
(c) Find a length x_0 of a fish such that 25% of the fish are shorter than x_0.

Solutions: Let X be the length of a fish from this cohort. We have $X \sim N(40, 3^2)$.

(a) The percentage of fish from this cohort that are longer than 45 cm is

$$\begin{aligned}P(X > 45) &= 1 - P(X \le 45)\\ &= 1 - \Phi\left(\frac{45-40}{3}\right)\\ &= 1 - \Phi(1.67) = 1 - 0.9525 = 0.0475.\end{aligned}$$

(b) The probability that a randomly selected fish from this cohort is between 37 cm and 43 cm is equal to

$$\begin{aligned}P(37 < X < 43) &= \Phi\left(\frac{43-40}{3}\right) - \Phi\left(\frac{37-40}{3}\right)\\ &= \Phi(1.00) - \Phi(-1.00)\\ &= 0.8413 - 0.1587 = 0.6826.\end{aligned}$$

(c) Solving and using Table 17.2

$$0.25 = P(X < x_0) = \Phi\left(\frac{x_0 - 40}{3}\right),$$

we get $(x_0 - 40)/3 = -0.675$. Thus, 25% of the fish are shorter than $x_0 = -0.675(3) + 40 = 37.975$ cm. (From Table 17.2, we use the fact that $\Phi(-0.67) = 0.2514$ and $\Phi(-0.68) = 0.2483$. Since 0.25 is between 0.2483 and 0.2514, we take the midpoint between -0.67 and -0.68, i.e. we use the fact that $\Phi(-0.675) = 0.25$.)

7.3 Problems

Problem 7.1. Suppose that the height of an 8-year old boy has a normal distribution with a mean of 125 cm and standard deviation of 8 cm.
(a) What is the probability that a randomly chosen 8-year old boy is shorter than 122 cm?
(b) What is the probability that a randomly chosen 8-year old boy has a height between 122 cm and 130 cm?
(c) We would like to say that 95% of the 8-year old boys have a height smaller than h. What is the value h?

Problem 7.2. The blue whale is a marine mammal belonging to the suborder of baleen whales and is the largest animal ever known to have existed on Earth. Assuming that the length of a blue whale is a normally distributed random variable with a mean of 33 m and standard deviation of 4 m, find the percentage of blue whales that have a length larger than 35 m.

Problem 7.3. The growth of a tomato seedling in a month is a normal random variable X with the mean of 2 cm and the standard deviation of 0.7 cm.
(a) What is the probability that a seedling does not germinate (i.e. $X \leq 0$)?
(b) In a greenhouse, tomato seedlings are arranged in trays of 25 small compartments each, with one seedling planted in each compartment. Such a tray is randomly selected. What is the probability that in this tray, all compartments contain seedlings which did germinate?

Problem 7.4. Let Z be a standard normal random variable. Use Table 17.2 and Table 17.3 to compute the following probabilities:
(a) $P(Z > 1.96)$ (b) $P(Z < -0.05)$ (c) $P(1.1 < Z < 2.5)$
(d) $P(Z < 0.96)$ (e) $P(Z > -2.35)$ (f) $P(-2.23 < Z < 2.23)$.
If you have access to a statistical package, use the computer to find the above probabilities, and compare these values with the answers obtained using the tables.

Problem 7.5. Let X be a normal random variable with a mean of 100 and a standard deviation of 36. Use Table 17.2 and Table 17.3 to compute the following probabilities :
(a) $P(X > 105)$ (b) $P(X < 98)$ (c) $P(93.5 < X < 112)$
(d) $P(X < 121.5)$ (e) $P(X > 90)$ (f) $P(82.5 < X < 117.5)$.
(Use rounding to 2 decimal places.) If you have access to a statistical package, use the computer to find the above probabilities, and compare these values with the answers obtained using the tables.

Problem 7.6. Assume that X is a normal random variable with a mean of 100 and a standard deviation of 36. Use Table 17.2 and Table 17.3 to find x_0 such that
(a) $P(X > x_0) = 0.05$ (b) $P(X < x_0) = 0.05$
(c) $P(-x_0 < X - 100 < x_0) = 0.95$ (d) $P(X < x_0) = 0.90$
(e) $P(X > x_0) = 0.99$ (f) $P(|X - 100| > 6\,x_0) = 0.05$.
If you have access to a statistical package, use the computer to find the above quantities, and compare these values with the answers obtained using the tables.

Problem 7.7. Blood pressure is a measure of the blood force against the walls of the arteries. The larger value represents the pressure when the heart contracts and pushes blood out (systolic), and the smaller value is the lowest pressure when the heart relaxes between beats (diastolic). Blood pressure that is consistently more than 140/90 mm Hg is considered high, but for

people with diabetes, 130/80 mm Hg is considered high. Normal blood pressure is below 120/80 mm Hg (source: http://www.heartandstroke.com). Consider a population of non-diabetic males with a mean systolic blood pressure of 115 mm Hg, in which 19% are classified as having high blood pressure (i.e. more than 140 mm Hg). Assume that the systolic blood pressure X is normally distributed.
(a) Compute the standard deviation of the systolic blood pressure of X.
(b) Compute the median, the first quartile and the third quartile of X. Hint: The median of X is the value a for which $P(X < a) = 0.5$. The first and third quartiles of X are the values b and c for which $P(X < b) = 0.25$, respectively $P(X < c) = 0.75$.
(c) The authors of [13] define stage 1 hypertension as a systolic blood pressure between 140 mm Hg and 160 mm Hg, or a diastolic blood pressure between 90 mm Hg and 100 mm Hg. Compute the probability that a randomly selected individual from this population is classified as having stage 1 hypertension according to the value of the systolic blood pressure, ignoring the value of the diastolic blood pressure.
(d) Stage 2 hypertension is defined as a systolic blood pressure larger than 160 mm Hg, or a diastolic blood pressure larger than 100 mm Hh. Compute the probability that a randomly selected individual from this population is classified as having stage 2 hypertension according to the value of the systolic blood pressure, ignoring the value of the diastolic blood pressure.

Problem 7.8. The grizzly bear (*Ursus arctos horribilis*) is a large animal which generally lives in the uplands of western North America. Its weight is dependent on location. It is estimated that an adult male grizzly bear from the Alaska Peninsula region has a mean weight of 357 kg with a standard deviation of 21 kg (see [51]). Assume that the weight of an adult male grizzly bear is normally distributed.
(a) What is the probability that an adult male grizzly bear from the Alaska Peninsula region weighs more than 420 kg?
(b) What is the probability that an adult male grizzly bear from the Alaska Peninsula region weighs more than 300 kg?
(c) Find a weight x_0 (in kg) such that 5% of the adult male grizzly bears from the Alaska Peninsula region weigh less than x_0.
(d) Find a weight y_0 (in kg) such that 75% of the adult male grizzly bears from the Alaska Peninsula region weigh less than y_0.
(e) If we select 6 adult male grizzly bears from the Alaska Peninsula region, what is the probability that at most 2 weigh less than 300 kg?

Did you know that? *The fact that the Earth is spherical in shape was first suggested by the Greek philosophers in the 6th century B.C., out of mysticism, and rationalized by Aristotle in the 4th century B.C. This fact became widely accepted after Magellan's expedition around the world (1519-1522). However, the fact that the Earth has an equatorial bulge (and thus, is not a prefect sphere) became the subject of a scientific controversy in the 17th century. First pointed out by Isaac Newton, and later contested by a French astronomer named Jean Cassini, the existence of the equatorial bulge was proved in 1735 by two French expeditions, who made precise measurements of the curvature of the Earth's surface, near the Equator, and near the North Pole. These expeditions proved that the equatorial bulge is 13 miles high at sea level. The difficulties encountered by these two expeditions triggered a much needed reform in the standard of measurements, which led to the establishment of the metric system by the French scientists in 1795. More details about this story can be found in* [6].

Chapter 8

Supplementary Problems (Probability)

Problem 8.1. Consider the RNA sequence GGGAAACCC. Since GGG is the code for glycine (*gly*), AAA is the code for lysine (*lys*) and CCC is the code for proline (*pro*), this sequence is one of the possible codes for *gly-lys-pro*. There are 4 synonyms for glycine, (GGG, GGC, GGU, GGA) 2 synonyms for lysine (AAA, AAG), and 4 synonyms for proline (CCC, CCU, CCA, CCG). How many codes are for *gly-lys-pro*?

Problem 8.2. A woman and a man have type A, respectively type B blood, but they do not know their genotypes.
(a) List all the possible cases of genotype crosses for this couple.
(b) In each of the cases listed in (a), construct the Punnett square which gives all the possible genotypes and phenotypes of their offspring.
(c) Is it possible that their offspring has type O blood? Justify your answer using (b).

Problem 8.3. One of the common symptoms of Alzheimer's disease is the memory loss that disrupts daily life. This is just one of the 10 warning signs of Alzheimer's disease. Another frequently encountered sign consists in having difficulty to complete familiar tasks. In a large group of early stage Alzheimer patients, 85% of them experience memory loss, 78% have difficulty completing familiar tasks and 67% show both signs.
(a) What is the probability that an early stage Alzheimer patient shows one of these signs?
(b) What is the probability that an early stage Alzheimer patient does not show any of these two signs?

Problem 8.4. Due to massive hunting, the grey wolves were considered an endangered species at the end of the 20th century. In 1995, 14 wolves

from Canada were reintroduced in the Yellowstone National Park, followed by 17 wolves the next year. The reintroduction program was so successful that today the wolf population in the United States is estimated at 4,500. Despite its success, the program is highly criticized, due to the loss of livestock in the affected regions. In a survey conducted on 850 participants which included 250 farmers and 600 non-farmers, 189 farmers and 433 non-farmers said that they would like to see a significant increase in the wolf hunting quota in their states.
(a) Using the data from this survey, estimate the percentage of people who are in favor of an increase in the wolf hunting quota.
(b) What is the probability that a randomly selected person in the affected regions is not in favor of an increase in the wolf hunting quota?

Problem 8.5. According to recent estimates, only 45% of people in Africa have access to safe drinking water, this being the major cause of many waterborne diseases. The incidence rate of waterborne diseases in communities which do not have access to safe drinking water is 88%, whereas in communities which do have access to safe drinking water, this rate is 32%.
(a) What is the incidence rate of waterborne diseases in Africa?
(b) A patient suffering from a waterborne disease is randomly chosen from a clinic in an African village. What is the probability that this patient did not have access to safe drinking water?

Problem 8.6. Rheumatoid arthritis (RA) is a chronic inflammatory disease that affects synovial joints. About 1% of the world's population suffers from this disease. A serological test for the presence of the anti-citrullinated protein antibodies is commonly used when rheumatoid arthritis is suspected. This test is positive in a proportion of 67% of all RA cases, and is negative 95% of the times when RA is not present.
(a) What is the sensitivity and the specificity of the test?
(b) What is the positive predicted value and the negative predictive value of the test?

Problem 8.7. (a) A lab has a population of 25 fruit flies, of which 5 are black and 20 are grey. A sample of 2 flies is selected. Is the fact that the second selected fly is black independent of the first one being black?
(b) Suppose now that there are 10,000 flies in the lab, of which 2,000 are black and 8,000 are grey. A sample of 2 flies is selected. Is the fact that the second selected fly is black independent of the first one being black?

Problem 8.8. According to a 2004 World Health Organization report, the average number of cases of leukemia in Canada is 6 per 100,000 habitants. Assume that the number of cases of leukemia has a Poisson distribution. What is the probability that among 10,000 people, there is at least one person who has leukemia?

Problem 8.9. Hemophilia is a genetic disorder which impairs the body's ability to control blood clotting. People affected by this disorder may have external or internal bleedings. It is estimated that 1 in 10,000 people suffer from hemophilia. Assume that the number of hemophilia cases follows a Poisson distribution.
(a) What is the average number of cases in the Canadian population of 35,260,000 habitants (as of September 2010)?
(b) What is the probability that in a community of 15,000 people, there are at least two cases of hemophilia?

Problem 8.10. The latest census of the mountain gorilla in the Virunga National Park (Congo) was completed in 2010. When counting mountain gorilla, primatologists try to avoid the direct contact with the animals, and rely instead on fecal samples. Suppose that in a given day, a team of primatologists will collect and analyze fecal samples until they have one of each sex, or a maximum of three samples.
(a) Let X be the number of fecal samples collected in one day. Give the probability mass function of X. Calculate the expected value of X.
(b) Let Y be the number of female fecal samples collected in one day. Give the probability mass function of Y. Calculate the expected value of Y.

Problem 8.11. Consider a research group of 6 professors and 20 students. A committee must be formed, consisting of 3 professors and 5 students.
(a) In how many ways can we select the members of this committee?
(b) One of the three selected professors will occupy the position of chairperson. In how many different ways can we select the members of this committee, including the assignment of the chairperson?

Problem 8.12. Twenty volunteers take part in an experiment. We would like to split them into five equally-sized treatment groups, each group being assigned a different treatment. This is called a balanced experimental design.
(a) In how many different ways can we accomplish this task? Hint: Break down the assignment of the subjects to treatment groups into steps and use the multiplication principle.
(b) Only four of the volunteers are over the age of sixty. We would like

to separate the older volunteers so that they are in four different groups. In how many different ways can we divide the twenty volunteers into the five treatment groups, if the four older volunteers must be in four different groups?

Problem 8.13. Consider a large lake in which 23% of the fish have tumors, 5% of the fish are young, and 0.5% of the fish are young and have tumors. What is the probability that a randomly chosen fish from this lake
(a) is young or has tumors?
(b) is young but does not have tumors?
(c) has tumors but is not young?

Problem 8.14. A blood donation center has been collecting data for many years. They noticed that 1% of all donors are positive for HIV and 2% are positive for herpes. If 1.5% of all donors are positive for only one of these conditions (but not both), what is the probability that a randomly chosen donor has none of these two conditions?

Problem 8.15. Refer to Problem 4.7 and Problem 4.8. A person is randomly selected from this country. Let A be the event that the person is infected with HIV and B be the event that the person is infected with tuberculosis. Are the events A and B mutually exclusive? Are the events A and B independent?

Problem 8.16. Assume that the probability that a child is a girl is 0.5. A couple has 3 children.
(a) What is the probability that all three children are girls?
(b) Given that the oldest and the youngest are girls, compute the probability that all children are girls.
(c) Compute the probability that at least one child is a girl.

Problem 8.17. The authors of [63] discuss an outbreak of schistosomiasis in brant geese (*Branta Bernicla Hrota*). They conjecture that the translocation of the geese from their natural environment to a pond may have caused them to be exposed to parasites. Suppose that 5% of the geese in a particular region are infected with schistosomiasis. 5 geese are randomly selected from this region.
(a) Compute the expected number of geese that do not have a schistosomiasis infection.
(b) Calculate the probability that at least one of the geese does not have a schistosomiasis infection.

PART 2
Statistics

Chapter 9

Introduction to Statistics

Statistics is one of the oldest disciplines in science, whose origins can be traced back to the 17th century when the British administration needed a tool for analyzing various demographic and economical data. The scope of the discipline became larger in the 19th century to include the analysis of data in general. Today, statistics is employed by people working in diverse fields, like economics, engineering, social sciences, and natural sciences.

In this chapter, we discuss several methods for analyzing data, using numerical summaries and graphical tools. We emphasize the distinction between a population and a random sample from a population. We explain how a random sample can be used to estimate population parameters, and discuss ways to measure the estimation error. Finally, we end this chapter with a discussion on the sampling distribution of estimators, which includes an introduction to the T distribution. We also give the Central Limit Theorem which states that the distribution of a sample mean can be approximated by a normal distribution.

9.1 Random Sampling and Data Description

In this section, we learn to describe data using numerical summaries (called descriptive statistics) and graphical representations. We consider the data as observations from a random variable. The set of these observations is called a *random sample*. The techniques that we use to describe the sample depend on the variable type.

If the values of the variable represent categories, then we say that the variable is *categorical*. The table below contains examples of categorical variables.

Variable	Categories
colour of pee pod	yellow, green
type of fish	Northern pike, Rainbow trout, Catfish
height	small, medium, large

A variable is called *quantitative* (or *numerical*) if it represents a numerical quantity. Temperature (in Kelvin), surface area in (cm^2), volume (in m^3), height (in cm), and number of diseased individuals, are examples of quantitative variables.

For categorical variables an easy and effective way to describe the data is to display a *frequency distribution* or a *relative frequency distribution.* When defining the categories one has to be careful in defining mutually exclusive classes, otherwise the relative frequencies do not add up to 1. The (relative) frequency distribution can be displayed as a table, or graphically, as a bar chart.

Example 9.1. A fish tumour survey was conducted in a particular river system. Of particular interest were liver tumours and tumours in the mouth. A random sample of $n = 123$ fish were captured, classified and released. The frequency distribution is displayed below in tabular form and as a bar chart in Figure 9.1.

Tumour Classification	Frequency	Relative Frequency
only liver	35	28.5%
only mouth	10	8.1%
both	3	2.4%
no tumours	75	61.0%
total	123	100%

Many biological studies are comparative in nature. These studies usually involve two or more variables. In the case of two categorical variables, we can start by cross-classifying the observations according to the joint categories of the two variables. The resulting table is called a contingency table and it displays the *joint (relative) frequency distribution* of the two variables.

To describe the association between the two variables, we can compute *conditional relative frequency distributions* for one of the variables conditioned on the categories of the other variables. The conditional relative frequency distribution can be displayed as a side-by-side bar chart.

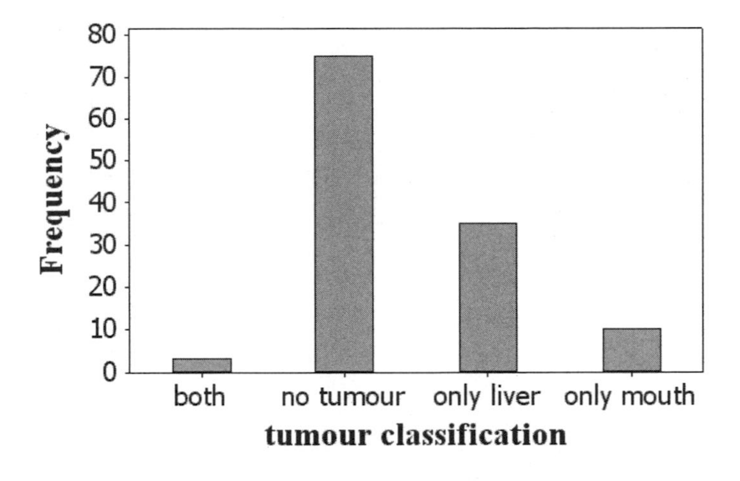

Fig. 9.1 Distribution of fish tumours

Example 9.2. Consider a fish tumour survey similar to Example 9.1. We would like to compare the fish tumour distributions in two river systems. A summary of the data is found in the following contingency table, which is a cross-classification of the fish according to the tumour category and the river systems. Each cell represents a joint frequency. In the parenthesis, we computed the conditional relative frequency for the tumour variable conditioned on the river system.

River	Tumour Category				
System	only liver	only mouth	both	no tumour	Total
1	35 (28.5%)	10 (8.1%)	3 (2.4%)	75 (61%)	123
2	15 (5.36%)	8 (2.86%)	2 (0.71%)	255 (91.07%)	280

In Figure 9.2, we find a side-by-side bar chart of the conditional distributions for tumour. The distribution of tumours do appear to be heterogeneous. In fact, it appears that fish from the second river system are more likely to have no tumours.

The frequency distribution is an important tool to describe the random sample from a quantitative variable. The frequency distribution can be displayed in tabular form, or with a graphical display called a *histogram.*

To construct the histogram of the frequency distribution, we divide the range of the sample into intervals of equal width (called *bins*). To build the

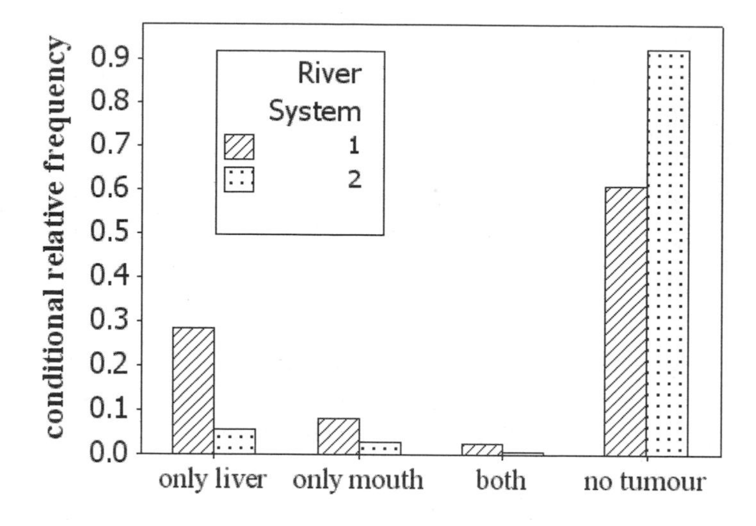

Fig. 9.2 Conditional distribution of fish tumours

histogram we erect a rectangle for each bin, whose height can be either the frequency (in the case of a frequency histogram) or the relative frequency (in the case of a relative frequency histogram). If the bins are of equal length, then the area of the rectangle is proportional to the relative frequency. We can also produce a probability density histogram, in which the height of the rectangle is equal to the relative frequency divided by the length of the interval. For a probability density histogram, the area of each rectangle is equal to the relative frequency.

When constructing a histogram with unequal bins, we suggest to use a probability density histogram. Otherwise, the area of the rectangles are not necessarily proportional to the relative frequency. This means that some values may appear to be more likely than they actually are.

There exist different rules for the number of bins to use in a histogram. A rule that usually works well is to use between 5 and 20 bins. Moreover, the number of bins should be approximately equal to $\sqrt{n}$, where n is the sample size. The use of a statistical package is recommended for producing the graphs. For most statistical packages, the default number of bins works well.

Example 9.3. Consider the following data, which gives the clutch sizes for

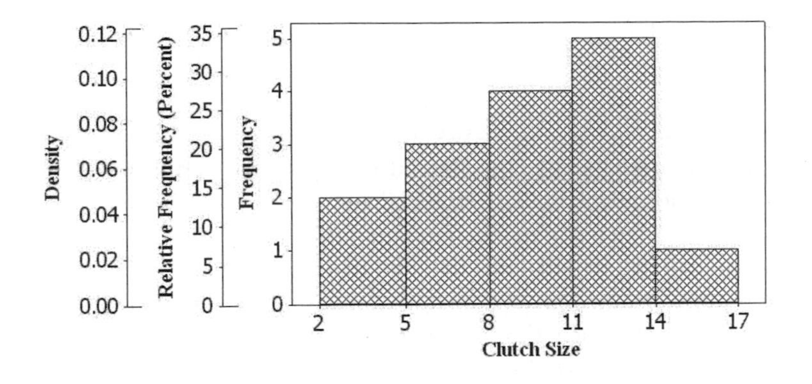

Fig. 9.3 Histogram of clutch size

$n = 15$ mallards for a particular region and year.

11	12	11	9	11	2	6	3
17	6	10	10	8	11	5	

To build the frequency distribution, we partition the range of the sample into 5 bins of equal length. For each bin, we compute the frequency, relative frequency and probability density. Using the frequency distribution, we produce the corresponding histogram (see Figure 9.3). The distribution of the clutch sizes appears to be slightly skewed to the left.

x = clutch size	frequency	relative frequency	probability density
$2 \leq x < 5$	2	$2/15 = 13.33\%$	$(2/15)/3 = 0.0444$
$5 \leq x < 8$	3	$3/15 = 20\%$	$(3/15)/3 = 0.0667$
$8 \leq x < 11$	4	$4/15 = 26.67\%$	$(4/15)/3 = 0.0889$
$11 \leq x < 14$	5	$5/15 = 33.33\%$	$(5/15)/3 = 0.1111$
$14 \leq x \leq 17$	1	$1/15 = 6.67\%$	$(1/15)/3 = 0.0222$

To describe properly the frequency distribution of a quantitative variable, we consider its shape, central tendencies and dispersion.

Below are examples of histograms that are approximately symmetric, skewed to the right, or skewed to the left, respectively. The *skewness* is the direction of the atypical values.

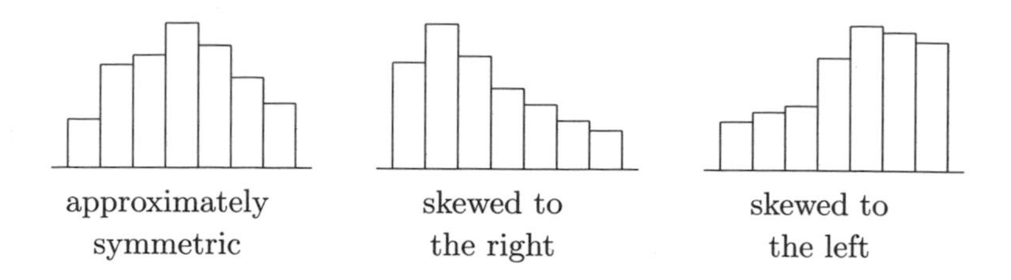

Before presenting different descriptive measures of central tendency and dispersion, we introduce the notion of sample quantiles. Quantiles are values that allow us to divide the ordered data into approximately equal-sized data subsets.

A quantile that divides the sample into two approximately equal-sized data subsets is called a *median*. One way to obtain a median $\tilde{x}$ for the sample $x_1, \ldots, x_n$ is to put the sample values in ascending order $y_1 \leq y_2 \leq \cdots \leq y_n$ and compute

$$\tilde{x} = \begin{cases} y_{\{(n+1)/2\}}, & \text{if } n \text{ is odd} \\ (y_{\{n/2\}} + y_{\{n/2+1\}})/2, & \text{if } n \text{ is even.} \end{cases}$$

Example 9.3 (Continued). Since the sample size $n = 15$ is odd, then the $(n+1)/2 = 8$th value in the ordered sample is a median. We arrange the data in ascending order as follows:

2	3	5	6	6	8	9	10
10	11	11	11	11	12	17	

So $\tilde{x} = 10$ is a median for this sample.

Quantiles that divide the sample into four approximately equal-sized data subsets are called *quartiles*. There are three quartiles that we denote as $q_1, q_2 = \tilde{x}, q_3$ for the first, second and third quartile, respectively. Note that the second quartile is the median.

One way to obtain the first quartile q_1 for the sample $x_1, \ldots, x_n$ is to put the sample values in ascending order $y_1 \leq y_2 \leq \cdots \leq y_n$. Compute $(n+1)/4$ and represent this quantity as a whole part r and a fractional part a/b. For example, for $n = 14$, we get $(n+1)/4 = 3.75$. The whole part is $r = 3$ and fractional part is $a/b = 0.75$. If the fractional part is zero, then r is the rank of the first quartile. If the fractional part is not zero, then the first quartile is a weighted average of the rth and the $(r+1)$th ordered value. We compute the first quartile as follows:

$$q_1 = \begin{cases} y_r, & \text{if } a/b = 0 \\ (1 - a/b)\, y_r + (a/b)\, y_{r+1}, & \text{if } a/b \neq 0. \end{cases}$$

For the third quartile, the computation is the same, except that we compute its rank as follows $(3/4)(n+1) = r + a/b$.

Example 9.3 (Continued). The rank of the first quartile is $(15+1)/4 = 4.0$. Hence the first quartile is the 4th ordered value, that is $q_1 = y_4 = 6$. The third quartile is $q_3 = y_{12} = 11$.

There is no uniquely accepted way to compute quantiles. In Example 9.3 any value between 5 and 6 could be used as a first quartile, since approximately 25% of the observations in the sample are smaller than it. Therefore, different statistical packages can produce different quantiles. However, for large samples sizes, the differences are often not significant.

To describe the central tendencies and dispersion of the sample, it is often useful to produce the following *5-number summary*: the minimum and maximum values, and the three quartiles. For Example 9.3, the 5-number summary is

$$\min = y_1 = 2, \ q_1 = 6, \ \tilde{x} = 10, \ q_3 = 11, \ \max = y_n = 17.$$

The median $\tilde{x} = 10$ can be used as measure of central tendency. A natural measure of dispersion is the *sample range*

$$R = y_n - y_1.$$

The sample range is considered as a rough measure of dispersion since it is based on the most extreme values in the sample. To obtain another measure of dispersion (that is not based on the extremes), we consider the *interquartile range*

$$\mathsf{IQR} = q_3 - q_1.$$

For Example 9.3, $\mathsf{IQR} = 11 - 6 = 5$.

A graphical display that goes hand-in-hand with the 5-number summary is called a *box plot* (or a *box-and-whisker plot*). This is a useful tool to display the center and dispersion of the data, and can be used to identify departures from symmetry and outlying values. Side-by-side box plots are also useful to compare two or more distributions, as we will see in Example 9.4.

To construct the box plot, extend the box from the first quartile to the third quartile. The box displays the interquartile range. Within the box, display a line at the median. Imaginary fences are placed at a distance of 1.5 IQR above the third quartile and below the first quartile. Whiskers extend from the ends of the box to the smallest and the largest values within the imaginary fences. Values outside the fences are called *outliers.* Each outlier is displayed as a point. Sometimes a different symbol is used for extreme outliers that are at least 3 IQR above q_3 or below q_1.

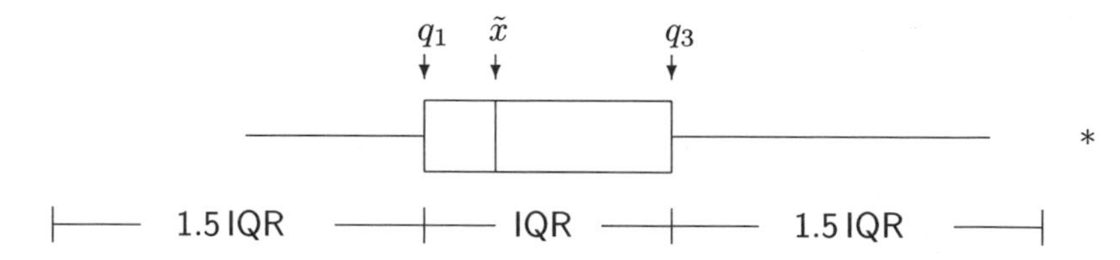

Example 9.4. We use side-by-side box plots to compare the distribution of the mallard clutch sizes from Example 9.3 to the following sample which are mallard clutch sizes from a different region.

6	7	8	8	8	9	9	9	9	9
10	10	10	10	10	10	10	11	12	14

For this data set, $n = 20$, $\tilde{x} = (y_{10} + y_{11})/2 = 9.5, q_1 = (0.75)\, y_5 + (0.25)\, y_6 = 8.25$, $q_3 = (0.25)\, y_{15} + (0.75)\, y_{16} = 10$ and $\mathsf{IQR} = 1.75$. The box plots are given in Figure 9.4. The samples appear to have similar central tendencies. The clutch sizes from the second region are less dispersed compared to the first region. Furthermore, the clutch size of 14 in sample 2 is an outlier when compared to other clutch sizes from the same region, since it exceeds the fence located at $q_3 + 1.5\,\mathsf{IQR} = 12.625$.

Another common measure for the central tendency of the distribution is the *sample mean* $\overline{x}$, defined as the arithmetic mean (also called the *average*) of the n observations:

$$x = \frac{x_1 + \ldots + x_n}{n} = \frac{\sum_{i=1}^{n} x_i}{n}.$$

If we put a mass of $1/n$ at the value x_i, then the sample mean can be interpreted as the centre of mass.

For symmetric or moderately skewed distributions, the mean is usually the preferred measure of central tendency since all values make a contribution to the mean. So why even bother with the median? The mean can be sensitive to extreme values, in the sense that the mean is pulled towards the extreme values. Hence the mean might not give an accurate representation

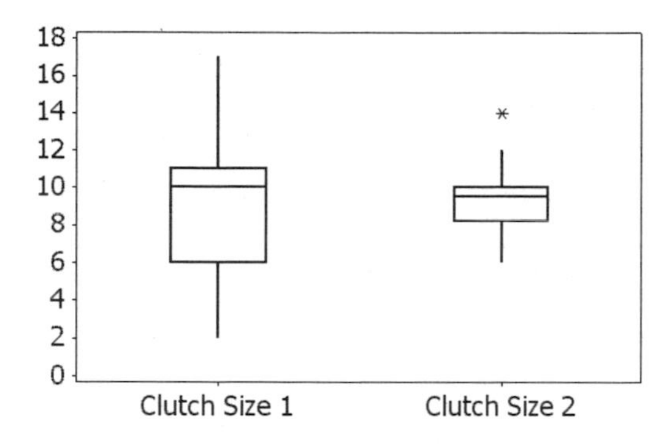

Fig. 9.4 Side-by-side boxplots

of the centre of the distribution in the presence of extreme values. Figure 9.5 illustrates this idea.

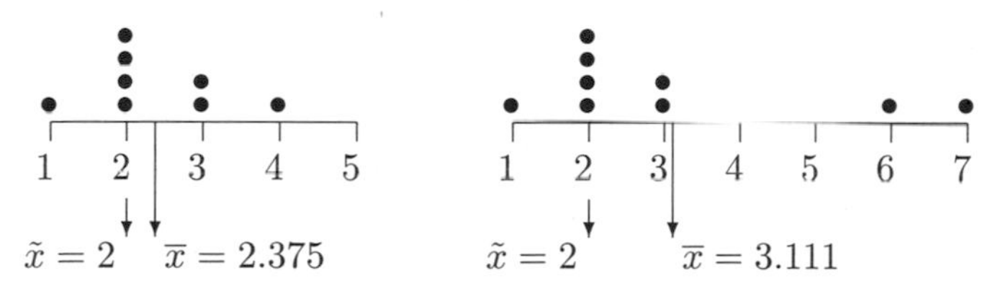

Fig. 9.5 Central tendencies

Since only the middle values make a contribution to the median, the median is insensitive to extreme values. This means that, for highly skewed distributions or distributions with extreme values, the median is often preferred over the mean as a measure of central tendency.

When the mean is used as a measure of the centre, we usually consider the sample variance and/or standard deviation as a measure of dispersion or variability. The *sample variance* is defined as

$$s^2 = \frac{\sum_{i=1}^{n}(x_i - \overline{x})^2}{n-1} = \frac{(\sum_{i=1}^{n} x_i^2) - (\sum_{i=1}^{n} x_i)^2/n}{n-1}.$$

The sample variance is approximately equal to the average squared deviation away from the mean. For a more dispersed distribution, the larger squared deviations away from the mean (on average) translate into a larger variance.

The variance is measured in squared units. To obtain a measure of dispersion measured in the same units as the variable, we compute the square root of the variance. The result is called the *sample standard deviation* and is denoted by s. Sometimes the mean and the standard deviation are combined to form an interval of one standard deviation about the mean: $\overline{x} \pm s$.

Example 9.5. Refer to the mallard clutch size Examples 9.3 and 9.4. For sample 1, the mean clutch size is $\overline{x}_1 = \sum_{i=1}^{15} x_i/15 = 132/15 = 8.8$ and the standard deviation for clutch size is

$$s_1 = \sqrt{\frac{(1372) - (132)^2/15}{15 - 1}} = 3.88.$$

So a typical clutch size in this region is between $\overline{x}_1 - s_1 = 8.8 - 3.88 = 4.92$ and $\overline{x}_1 + s_1 = 8.8 + 3.88 = 12.68$. Similar computations for sample 2, yield $\overline{x}_2 = 9.45$ and $s_2 = 1.731$. So a typical clutch size in the second region is between 7.719 and 11.181. The clutch sizes have a tendency to be larger in region 2 and are much less spread out. This is consistent with our description from Example 9.4.

Often scientists work with logarithmic units such as pH, decibels, and the Richter scale. Applying a logarithmic transformation can sometimes be useful when analyzing and describing data. If the frequency distribution is highly skewed to the right, then applying a logarithmic transformation to the observations changes the shape of the distribution. With a bit of luck, the distribution of the values on a logarithmic scale could be approximately symmetric. If so, then the mean and the standard deviation are meaningful measures of the center, respectively the spread of the distribution of the transformed variable. As we take the exponential of these statistics, we get the *geometric mean*:

$$g = e^{\overline{y}} = e^{\frac{1}{n}(\ln(x_1)+\ln(x_2)+\cdots+\ln(x_n))} = e^{\ln(x_1 x_2 \cdots x_n)^{1/n}} = (x_1 x_2 \cdots x_n)^{1/n}$$

and the *geometric standard deviation* e^{s_y}, where

$$s_y = \sqrt{\frac{1}{n-1}\sum_{i=1}^{n}(y_i - \overline{y})^2}$$

is the standard deviation of the natural log measurements $y_i = \ln x_i, i = 1, \ldots, n$. To summarize the geometric mean and the geometric standard deviation as an interval, we first construct the interval $\overline{y} \pm s_y$ of one standard deviation about the mean for the values $y_1, \ldots, y_n$ and then exponentiate. We get $g\, e^{\pm s_y} = [g/e^{s_y}, g\, e^{s_y}]$.

Example 9.6. Consider a sample of $n = 250$ survival times after the diagnosis of a particular type of cancer. The data is given in the file SurvivalTimes.txt. Typically, such survival time distributions are skewed to the right. We would like to describe the central tendencies and spread of these survival times. Figure 9.6 gives the histogram of the survival times in months. The mean is 16.24 months and the standard deviation is 21.46 months. The median is 9.45 months and the interquartile range is 13.45. The distribution is highly skewed and the mean is almost twice as large as the median.

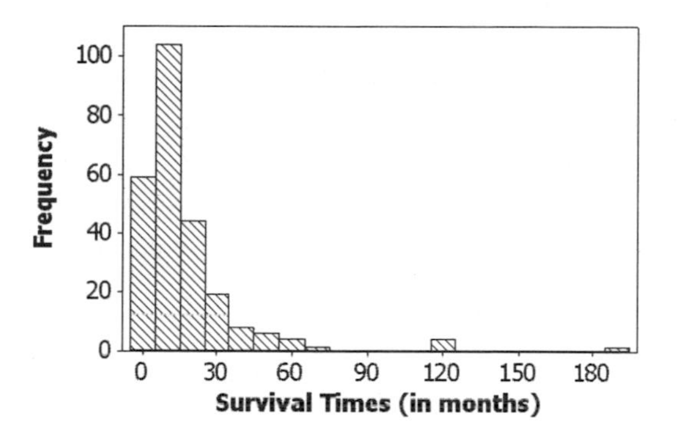

Fig. 9.6 Distribution of survival times

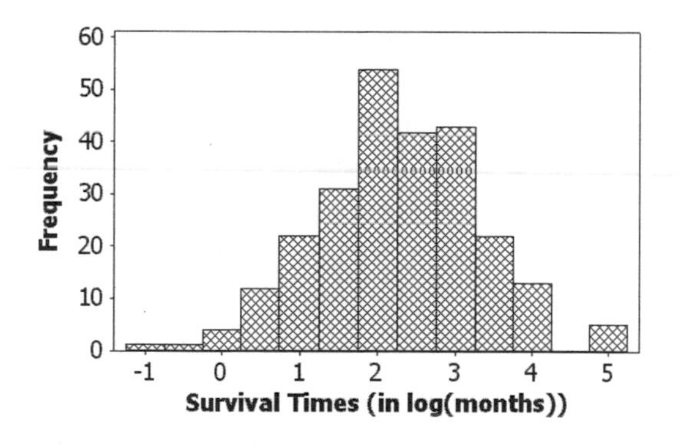

Fig. 9.7 Distribution of the log-survival times

Since the data is highly skewed, we apply a natural logarithm transformation to the observations, and produced the histogram in Figure 9.7. The distribution of the natural log-times appears to be approximately symmetric. Its mean is 2.2659 and its standard deviation is 1.0306. As we exponentiate the statistics of the log-values, we obtain measurements on the original scale. The results are a geometric mean of $g = e^{2.2659} = 9.64$ months and a geometric standard deviation of $e^{s_y} = 2.80$ months. So typical survival times are between $g/e^{s_y} = 3.44$ months and $g\, e^{s_y} = 26.99$ months.

We end this section with techniques that describe the association between two quantitative variables. We consider two examples. In Example 9.7, we describe the association between the heights of mothers and daughters. This is an example of a positive linear association, where the heights of the daughters tend to increase as the heights of the mothers increase. In Example 9.8, we examine the relationship between the number of colds and vitamin C. This is an example of a negative linear association. As the dosage of vitamin C increases, the number of colds tend to decrease on average.

Consider n paired observations (x_i, y_i), for $i = 1, \ldots, n$, from a pair (X, Y) of random variables. To describe the linear association between the two variables we use the *sample covariance*

$$s_{xy} = \frac{\sum_{i=1}^{n}(x_i - \overline{x})(y_i - \overline{y})}{n-1} = \frac{(\sum_{i=1}^{n} x_i\, y_i) - (1/n)(\sum_{i=1}^{n} x_i)(\sum_{i=1}^{n} y_i)}{n-1}.$$

If there is a positive linear association between X and Y, then for values x_i which are larger (respectively smaller) than $\overline{x}$, the corresponding y_i should tend to be larger (respectively smaller) than $\overline{y}$, which means that the covariance should be positive. However for a negative linear association, the values x_i which are larger (respectively smaller) than $\overline{x}$ will tend to correspond to values y_i that are smaller (respectively larger) than $\overline{y}$, which means that the covariance should be negative.

A better interpretation is obtained using an alternative statistic which is based on the covariance, called the *sample correlation*:

$$r_{xy} = \frac{s_{xy}}{s_x\, s_y},$$

where s_x and s_y are the respective sample standard deviations. The sample correlation is also called *Pearson's correlation*, or the *product-moment correlation*. The sample correlation satisfies the following properties which justify its suitability as a descriptive measure of linear association:

- It is invariant to linear scaling. In other words, the correlation remains the same regardless if we measure height in millimeters, centimeters or meters.
- It has the same sign as the covariance, so it is negative for negative linear associations and positive for positive linear associations.
- A correlation is always between -1 and 1. It is equal to 1 or -1 if and only if the points $(x_1, y_1), \ldots, (x_n, y_n)$ fall exactly on a line. Furthermore, if there is no association between X and Y, then the correlation should be near 0. In Section 15.1, we will learn how to interpret correlations that are not near 0 or ± 1, using a measure called the coefficient of determination.

CAUTION: If the relationship between X and Y is not linear, then the sample correlation is meaningless. In Section 15.2, we will see an example where there is a strong association between the two variables, but the correlation is near zero.

Example 9.7. The data below gives the heights (in cm) for a sample of $n = 12$ pairs of mother and daughter.

height						
daughter	160	165	156	169	152	156
mother	163	165	162	161	161	160
daughter	162	156	161	160	164	162
mother	164	159	164	161	163	168

Figure 9.8 gives the scatter plot of the height Y of the daughter against the height X of the mother. There appears to be a positive linear association between the two variables. The sample covariance is $s_{xy} = 4.9318$ and the respective standard deviations are $s_x = 2.4664$ and $s_y = 4.6928$. The sample correlation between the heights of the daughters and the mothers is equal to $r_{xy} = s_{xy}/(s_x\, s_y) = 0.426$.

Example 9.8. Consider an experiment where different daily dosages of vitamin C (in mg) were randomly assigned to subjects. For each subject, we count the number of times that the person contracted the common cold over a period of three years. Here are the data:

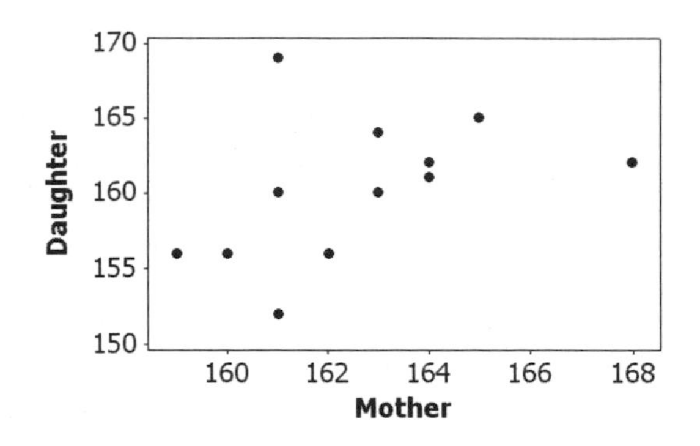

Fig. 9.8 Scatter plot for pairs of mother and daughter

Dosage (in mg)	Number of Colds				
0	12	10	10	15	14
15	14	7	8	11	9
30	10	12	9	8	11
50	7	10	8	4	6

Figure 9.9 gives the scatter plot of the number Y of colds against the daily dosage X of vitamin C. There appears to be a negative linear association between X and Y. The sample covariance is $s_{xy} = -34.0132$ and the respective standard deviations are $s_x = 18.9789$ and $s_y = 2.8074$. The sample correlation between the two variables is equal to $r_{xy} = -0.638$.

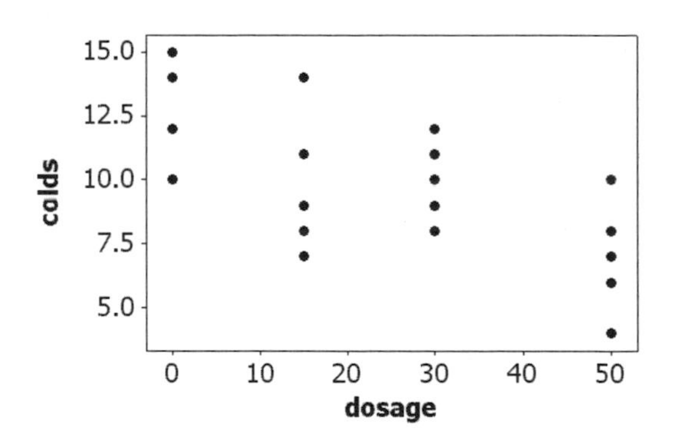

Fig. 9.9 Scatter plot: Number of colds against vitamin C

9.2 Sampling Distributions and Point Estimation

As part of the scientific method, scientists consider hypotheses that must be tested using experiments. This often involves making n independent measurements or drawing a random sample of size n. For example, we select n subjects and identify their blood type, or we select n small surfaces in a field and count the number of beetle larvae.

Definition 9.1. We model each observation as a random variable. We denote the random variable for the ith trial by X_i. We assume that the random variables are independent. If we repeat the same experiment at each trial, then we say that the random variables $X_1, X_2, \ldots, X_n$ are identically distributed. The common distribution is called the **population**. If $X_1, \ldots, X_n$ are independent and identically distributed, then we say that they are a **random sample** of size n from a particular population.

We are often interested in estimating some parameters of the population. Here are some examples of parameters.

- The mean μ of the population.
- The variance σ^2 (or the standard deviation σ) of the population.
- The proportion p of individuals in the population who have a certain characteristic.

To estimate a population parameter θ, we use a function of the random sample $X_1, \ldots, X_n$. This motivates the following definition:

Definition 9.2. A function of a random sample $X_1, \ldots, X_n$ is called a **statistic**. If the statistic

$$\widehat{\Theta} = h(X_1, X_2, \ldots, X_n)$$

is used to estimate the population parameter θ, then we say that $\widehat{\Theta}$ is a **point estimator** of θ. Note that $\widehat{\Theta}$ is a random variable since it is a function of random variables and it has a probability distribution. The probability distribution of a statistic is called a **sampling distribution**. The observed value of the random variable $\widehat{\Theta}$, which is $\widehat{\theta} = h(x_1, x_2, \ldots, x_n)$, is called a **point estimate** of θ.

Here are some common statistics:

- A point estimator for the population mean μ is the *sample mean* $\overline{X}$, defined as the average of $X_1, \ldots, X_n$:

$$\overline{X} = \frac{\sum_{i=1}^{n} X_i}{n}.$$

- A point estimator for the population variance is the *sample variance* S^2, defined as:
$$S^2 = \frac{\sum_{i=1}^n (X_i - \overline{X})^2}{n-1} = \frac{(\sum_{i=1}^n X_i^2) - (\sum_{i=1}^n X_i)^2/n}{n-1}.$$
- A point estimator for the population standard deviation is the *sample standard deviation* $S = \sqrt{S^2}$.
- A point estimator for the proportion p, is the *sample proportion* $\widehat{p}$, defined as:
$$\widehat{p} = \frac{Y}{n},$$
where Y is the number of individuals in the sample who have the desired characteristic, and n is the sample size.

Example 9.9. Consider the mallard clutch size data from Example 9.3. A point estimate for the mean clutch size of the population is $\hat{\mu} = \overline{x} = 8.8$ and a point estimate for the population standard deviation of the clutch size is $\widehat{\sigma} = \sqrt{s^2} = 3.88$. A point estimate for the population proportion p of clutches of size less than 6 is $\widehat{p} = y/n = 3/15 = 0.2$, where $y = 3$ represents the observed number of clutches less than 6 and $n = 15$ is the sample size.

Here is a summary of results concerning some properties of the expectation and variance. The results are used to study the properties of the estimators.

Theorem 9.1. *Consider random variables $X_1, X_2, \ldots, X_n$ and real constants $c_0, c_1, \ldots, c_n$. Let $Y = c_1 X_1 + \cdots + c_n X_n$, then*
$$E(Y) = c_1 E(X_1) + \cdots + c_n E(X_n).$$
Furthermore, if $X_1, X_2, \ldots, X_n$ are independent, then
$$\text{Var}(Y) = c_1^2 \text{Var}(X_1) + \cdots + c_n^2 \text{Var}(X_n).$$
As a special case, if X is a random variable, then
$$E(c_0 X) = c_0 E(X) \quad \text{and} \quad \text{Var}(c_0 X) = c_0^2 \text{Var}(X).$$

Example 9.10. Consider a random sample $X_1, \ldots, X_n$ from a population with mean μ and variance σ^2, that is $E(X_i) = \mu$ and $\text{Var}(X_i) = \sigma^2$, for $i = 1, \ldots, n$. Then,
$$\begin{aligned} E(\overline{X}) &= E\left(\frac{1}{n}X_1 + \cdots + \frac{1}{n}X_n\right) \\ &= \frac{1}{n}E(X_1) + \cdots + \frac{1}{n}E(X_n) \\ &= n\,\frac{1}{n}\mu = \mu \end{aligned}$$

and

$$\begin{aligned}\mathrm{Var}(\overline{X}) &= \mathrm{Var}\left(\frac{1}{n}X_1 + \cdots + \frac{1}{n}X_n\right) \\ &= \left(\frac{1}{n}\right)^2 \mathrm{Var}(X_1) + \cdots + \left(\frac{1}{n}\right)^2 \mathrm{Var}(X_n) \\ &= n\left(\frac{1}{n}\right)^2 \sigma^2 = \frac{\sigma^2}{n}.\end{aligned}$$

Example 9.11. Let Y denote the number of individuals who have a certain characteristic in a sample of size n. Since each individual has the same probability p of having this characteristic, Y has a binomial distribution with n trials and probability p of success. Let $\hat{p} = Y/n$. Then,

$$E(\hat{p}) = \frac{1}{n}E(Y) = \frac{1}{n}n\,p = p$$

and

$$\mathrm{Var}(\hat{p}) = \frac{1}{n^2}\mathrm{Var}(Y) = \frac{1}{n^2}n\,p\,(1-p) = \frac{p\,(1-p)}{n}.$$

When the expected value of an estimator is equal to the value of the parameter it is estimating, we say that the estimator is *unbiased*. Examples 9.10 and 9.11 show that the sample mean $\overline{X}$ is an unbiased estimator of the population mean μ, and the sample proportion $\widehat{p}$ is an unbiased estimator of the population proportion. It can also be shown that the sample variance S^2 is an unbiased estimator of the population variance σ^2.

Notice that $\mathrm{Var}(\overline{X})$ and $\mathrm{Var}(\widehat{p})$ become very small as the sample size becomes large. This means that, the probability distribution of the estimator becomes more concentrated about the value of the unknown parameter, as the sample size becomes larger.

When reporting an estimate it is important to give a measurement of the error. A common way to measure the error of the estimate is to use the standard deviation of the estimator. This is called the *standard error of the estimator.*

The standard error is often a function of some unknown parameters. If we substitute the unknown parameter with its point estimate, then we obtain the *estimated standard error*, that we denote by $s\{\widehat{\Theta}\}$. The estimated standard errors for the mean and the proportion are, respectively:

$$s\{\overline{X}\} = \frac{s}{\sqrt{n}} \quad \text{and} \quad s\{\widehat{p}\} = \sqrt{\frac{\widehat{p}\,(1-\widehat{p})}{n}}.$$

We end this section with a discussion on sampling distributions. We will see in the sections to follow that if we know (or approximately know) the sampling distribution of the estimator, we can construct interval estimates (called confidence intervals). These intervals give us a much better sense of the error of the estimate compared to the standard error.

Theorem 9.2. *Let $X_1, X_2, \ldots, X_n$ be independent normal random variables. Then $Y = c_1 X_1 + \cdots + c_n X_n$ is also a normal random variable.*

The normal distribution is often used as a model of the population. This assumption of normality is often reasonable. In Section 9.3, we will discuss some graphical techniques to verify this assumption. The next result says that if the population is normal, then the sample mean is also normally distributed.

Theorem 9.3. *Consider a random sample $X_1, \ldots, X_n$ from a normal population with mean μ and variance σ^2. As a consequence of Theorem 9.2, the sample mean $\overline{X}$ is normally distributed, that is*

$$\overline{X} = \frac{X_1 + \cdots + X_n}{n} \sim N\left(\mu, \sigma^2/n\right) \quad \textit{and} \quad \frac{\overline{X} - \mu}{\sigma/\sqrt{n}} \sim N(0, 1).$$

Note that in the standardization of the sample mean, we used the population standard deviation σ. Since σ is usually unknown, we will use the sample standard deviation S in its place. In this case, we call the standardization a *studentization*, which is

$$T = \frac{\overline{X} - \mu}{S/\sqrt{n}}.$$

Theorem 9.4. *If $X_1, \ldots, X_n$ is a random sample from a normal population, then the studentized variable T has a* ***T distribution*** *with $n - 1$ degrees of freedom. We denote this distribution by $T(n-1)$.*

In Figure 9.10, we have an overlay of the density for the T distribution for several degrees of freedom. The T distribution has a symmetric density similar to the standard normal, but it has heavier tails. In other words, the T distribution is more dispersed than the standard normal distribution. As the degrees of freedom increase, the T distribution gets more concentrated about the mean of zero. In fact, as the degrees of freedom become large, the T distribution approaches the standard normal distribution.

Table 17.4 gives the quantiles for the T distribution. For example, in the row for $\nu = 5$ degrees of freedom, we find the upper quantile $t_{0.05,\nu} = 2.015$.

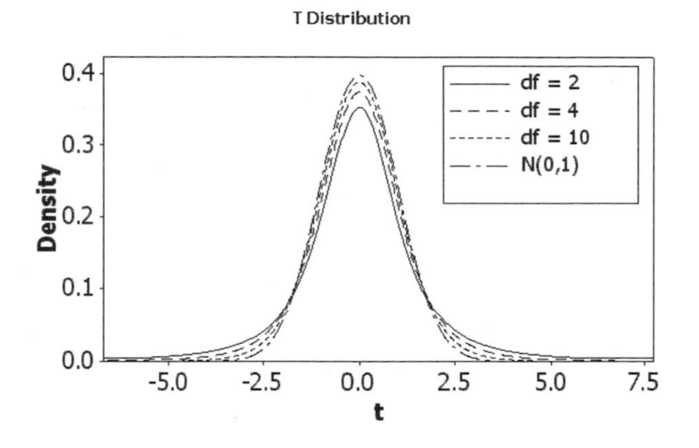

Fig. 9.10 Density for the T distribution for several degrees of freedom

Refer to Figure 9.11 for an illustration of this quantile. We interpret the quantile as follows: if T has a $T(5)$ distribution, then $P(T > 2.015) = 0.05$. Note that the table contains only positive quantiles. Since the distribution is symmetric, we can conclude that $P(T < -2.015) = 0.05$. So we can obtain probabilities associated to negative values by using a symmetry argument.

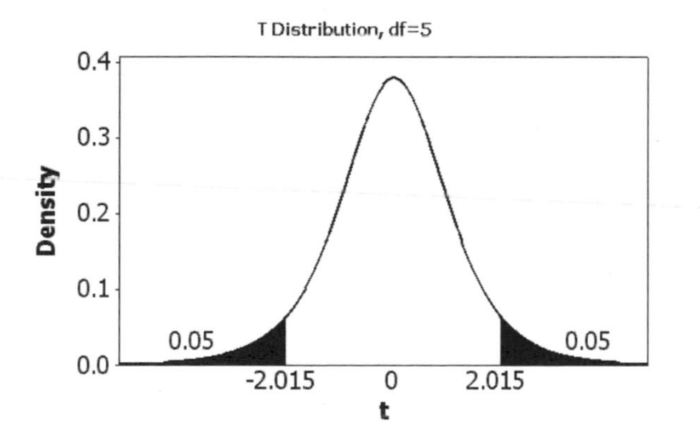

Fig. 9.11 A lower and upper quantile from the T distribution

Example 9.12. Suppose that the 14-day weight gain for a rat on a particular diet can be modeled as a normal random variable with a mean of 100 grams and a standard deviation of 30 grams. Suppose that we have a random sample of $n = 25$ such rats.

We would like to find the probability that the mean weight gain for these 25 rats is more than 110 grams. From Theorem 9.3, we know that the sample mean $\overline{X}$ follows a normal distribution with mean $\mu = 100$ grams and standard deviation $\sigma/\sqrt{n} = 30/\sqrt{25} = 6$ grams. Using the Standardization Theorem 7.1 and Table 17.3, we can compute the probability that the sample mean weight gain $\overline{X}$ is larger than 110 grams:

$$P(\overline{X} > 110) = 1 - \Phi\left(\frac{110 - 100}{6}\right) = 1 - \Phi(1.67) = 0.0475.$$

Note that $(110 - 100)/6 = 1.66667$, which we rounded to 1.67. Using a statistical software package, we obtain a more accurate answer: $P(\overline{X} > 110) = 0.04779035$.

We would like to find the probability that the studentization of the mean weight gain is less than -2.5. The studentization of the sample mean $\overline{X}$ is $T = (\overline{X} - \mu)/(S/\sqrt{n})$, which has a $T(24)$ distribution. We want to compute the probability $p = P(T < -2.5)$. We can compute this probability with a statistical software package. In this case the answer is $p = 0.009827$. We can alternatively use Table 17.4 to estimate this probability. First we start with a symmetry argument. Since the T distribution is symmetric about 0, $p = P(T > 2.5)$. We use the row for $\nu = 24$ degrees of freedom and try to find the quantiles closest to 2.5. We find $t_{0.01,24} = 2.492$ and $t_{0.005,24} = 2.797$. This means that $P(T > 2.492) = 0.01$ and $P(T > 2.797) = 0.005$. Thus, $0.005 < p < 0.01$.

Recall that the sampling distribution of the sample mean is normal when working with a random sample from a normal population, and its studentization follows a T distribution. Can we say anything concerning the sampling distribution of the sample mean in the case where the normal distribution is not a reasonable model for the population? Amazingly the answer is YES, as long as we have a large enough sample. More precisely, we have the following result:

Theorem 9.5. *Consider a random sample $X_1, \ldots, X_n$ from an unknown population with mean μ and variance σ^2. Consider the standardization and the studentization of the sample mean*

$$Z_n = \frac{\overline{X} - \mu}{\sigma/\sqrt{n}} \quad \text{and} \quad T_n = \frac{\overline{X} - \mu}{S/\sqrt{n}},$$

respectively. As $n \to \infty$, the limiting distribution of both Z_n and T_n is the standard normal.

The result for Z_n is known as the **Central Limit Theorem**. In essence, Theorem 9.5 says that we can use a normal approximation to compute probabilities associated with the sample mean:

$$P(\overline{X} \leq a) \approx \Phi\left(\frac{a-\mu}{\sigma/\sqrt{n}}\right).$$

How good is the normal approximation? Well, that depends on the shape of the population and the sample size. If the population is distributed normally, then the approximation is good even for small sample sizes. However, if the shape of the distribution is highly deviating from the normal distribution, then a larger sample size is required.

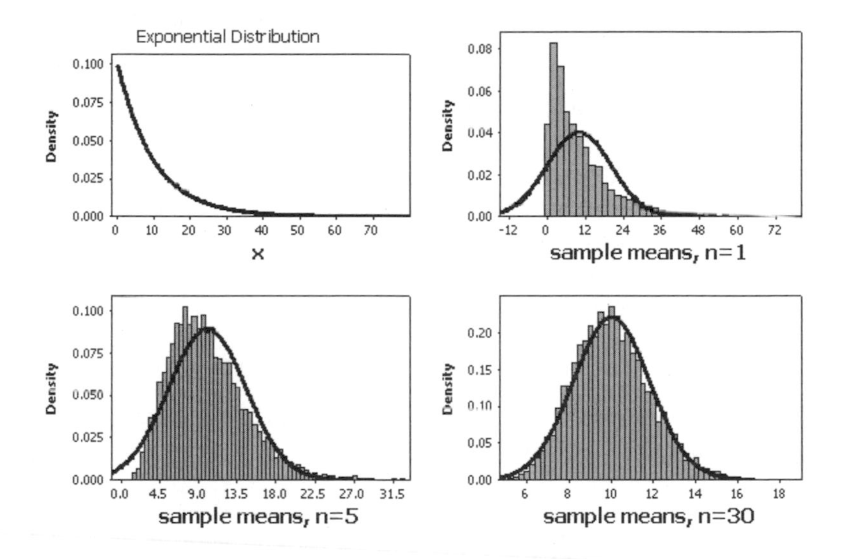

Fig. 9.12 Sampling distributions

To see the Central Limit Theorem in action, we use some computed generated data from an exponential distribution. Note that this density is highly skewed to the right, (see the upper left graph in Figure 9.12). We generated a random sample of size 5,000 and plotted the histogram. Each observation can be considered as a sample mean for a sample of size $n = 1$. We overlayed a normal density onto the histogram to compare the sampling distribution of the sample means of size $n = 1$ to a normal distribution. We see that the normal distribution does not fit the data very well (see the upper right graph in Figure 9.12).

To obtain the sampling distribution for the sample of size $n = 5$, we generated $n = 5$ observations from the same exponential distribution, and computed the mean. We replicated this process 5,000 times and plotted the 5,000 sample means of size $n = 5$. The result is in the lower left graph in Figure 9.12. We see that in this case there is a better fit between a normal distribution and the sampling distribution of the sample mean. However, the sampling distribution is still skewed to the right.

Finally, the same process was repeated in the lower right graph in Figure 9.12 to obtain the sampling distribution for the sample mean when $n = 30$. In this case, the sampling distribution appears to be approximately normal. This means that even though the population is highly skewed to the right, with a large enough sample, the sampling distribution of the sample mean is approximately normal.

Example 9.13. Suppose that we measure the growth of $n = 25$ plants that have been growing under certain conditions for a month. Suppose that such growth can be modeled as a random variable with a mean of 7 cm and a standard deviation of 1.5 cm. The approximate probability that the mean growth of the 25 plants is between 6 cm and 8 cm is

$$\begin{aligned} P(6 < \overline{X} < 8) &\approx \Phi\left(\frac{8-7}{1.5/\sqrt{25}}\right) - \Phi\left(\frac{6-7}{1.5/\sqrt{25}}\right) \\ &= \Phi(3.33) - \Phi(-3.33) = 0.9992. \end{aligned}$$

We used the fact that $\Phi(3.33) = 0.9996$ and $\Phi(-3.33) = 0.0004$ from Table 17.3 and Table 17.2, respectively.

9.3 Assessing Normality

In the next chapters, we will often use a normal distribution as a model of the true distribution for a variable. In this section we discuss techniques to assess the validity of such an assumption.

Both techniques that we discuss are visual in nature: the histogram, and the *quantile comparison plot* (or *QQ-plot*). We start the discussion with the histogram since we are familiar with it. If the variable is normally distributed then we should expect the shape of the histogram to be unimodal and symmetric. To help visualize the normal curve, we can overlay the probability density function of a normal random variable with the same mean and variance as the sample onto a density histogram.

Example 9.14. [Species Abundance] Species abundance is an index used to describe a biological community, and is defined as the number of individuals per species. We sampled $n = 500$ species in a particular forest. Figure 9.13 gives the histogram for the species abundance. The histogram is highly skewed. The species abundance does not appear to be normally distributed. Below is a summary of the data:

Species Abundance	Frequency	Species Abundance	Frequency
1	90	10	8
2	111	11	8
3	83	12	3
4	60	13	1
5	48	14	3
6	32	15	1
7	23	16	1
8	13	18	2
9	12	21	1

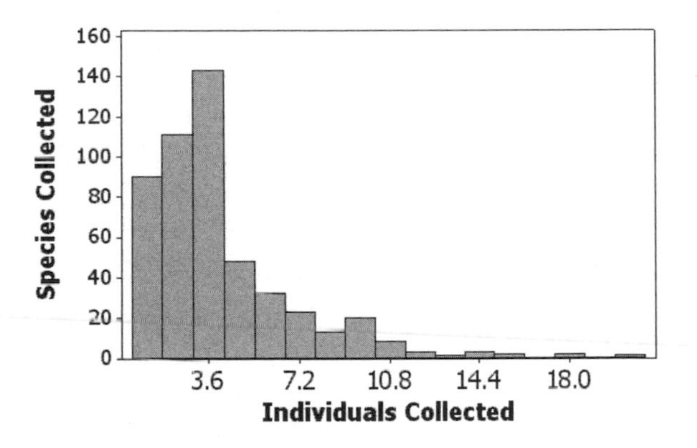

Fig. 9.13 Histogram for the species abundance

Another visual tool useful for assessing normality is called the *QQ-plot* (or a normal probability plot). Suppose that we can model the distribution of a random variable X with a normal distribution, that is $X \sim N(\mu, \sigma^2)$. By the Standardization Theorem 7.1,

$$Z = \frac{X - \mu}{\sigma} = \frac{1}{\sigma}X - \frac{\mu}{\sigma} \sim N(0, 1).$$

This show that there is a linear relationship between X and Z. If a sample $x_1, \ldots, x_n$ is generated from a normal distribution, then we should be able to observe this linear relationship.

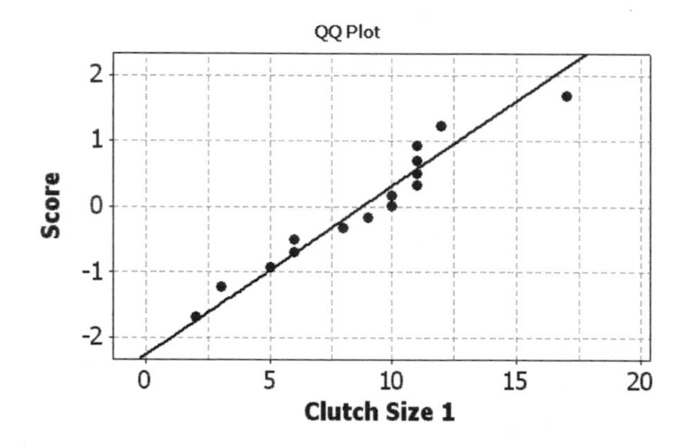

Fig. 9.14 QQ-plot for clutch size from Example 9.3

Suppose that we have a sample $x_1, \ldots, x_n$. The order statistics $y_1 \leq y_2 \leq \cdots \leq y_n$ are obtained by reordering the observations in ascending order. The *relative order* of the ith order statistic is defined as

$$p_i = \frac{i - 3/8}{n + 1/4}.$$

Consider the clutch size variable from Example 9.3. The value of the 3rd order statistic is $y_3 = 5$ which has a relative order of $p_3 = (3 - 3/8)/(15 + 1/4) = 0.172131$. This means that approximately 17.21% of the observations are smaller or equal to 5.

Let z_i be a quantile from the standard normal distribution of order p_i for $i = 1, \ldots, n$, i.e. z_i is a value such that $P(Z \leq z_i) = p_i$. We construct the QQ-plot by graphing the points (y_i, z_i) for $i = 1, \ldots, n$. If the data are normal, then there should be a linear tendency. To aid identify this linear tendency we can add the fitted line with slope $1/s$ and intercept $-\overline{x}/s$, where $\overline{x}$ and s are the sample mean and the sample standard deviation, respectively.

In Figure 9.14, we produced a QQ-plot for the clutch size from Example 9.3. Since the tendency in the QQ-plot appears to be linear, it is reasonable to use the normal distribution as a probability model for the clutch size.

There is a graph that is equivalent to the QQ-plot which is called a *normal probability plot*. Instead of displaying the score z_i, it is common practice to display the cumulative probability associated to z_i. Bear in mind that we should keep the scaling of the scores and not the scaling of the probabilities. In Figure 9.15, we constructed a normal probability plot for Species Abundance from Example 9.14. There appears to be a systematic tendency away from the normal curve, thus we have evidence against the normality of the species abundance.

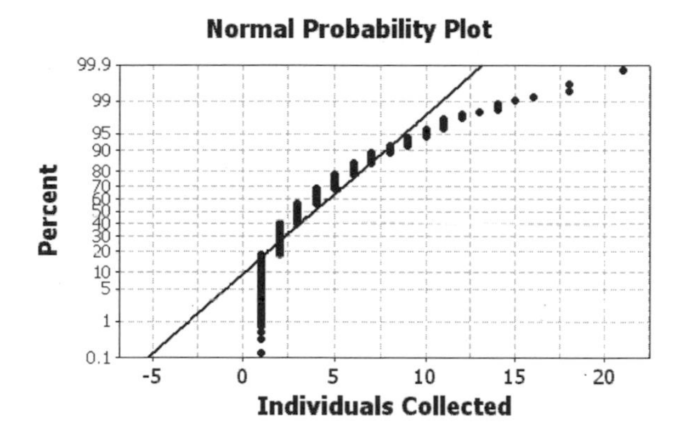

Fig. 9.15 Normal probability plot for the species abundance from Example 9.14

When comparing means from two or more independent populations, statisticians often make the assumption that the populations have an equal variance. A QQ-plot or normal probability plot can be used to verify this assumption of variance constancy. If we look closely at the slope of the linear relationship between the normal random variable X and the standard normal random variable Z, we see that it depends on the population standard deviation σ. Actually the slope is $1/\sigma$. The QQ-plots or normal probability plots of the two samples can be used to compare the variances.

Example 9.15. We study the effects of different irrigation methods on the yield of blueberry plants. Each method is assigned to 10 plots of blueberry plants. The yields (in kg) are below.

Irrigation Method 1									
7.3	6.5	9.4	7.2	8.4	5.5	5.6	9.7	4.5	5.3

Irrigation Method 2									
20.6	5.4	8.4	8.9	14.0	12.9	10.9	5.8	4.2	13.4

As we see in the side-by-side box plots in Figure 9.16, the yields for the different irrigation methods appear to have different variances. The second yield variable appears to be more dispersed. We can also compare the variances with a normal probability plot (see the right-hand-side in Figure 9.16). The fitted lines have different slopes which is further evidence that the variances of the yield variables are different.

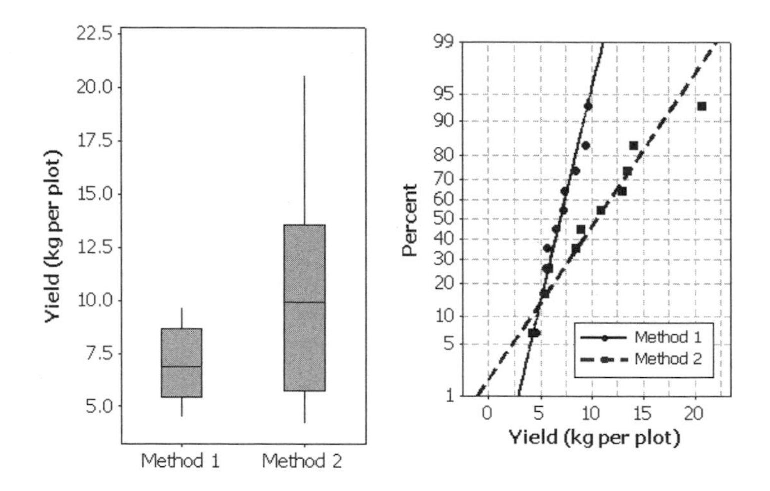

Fig. 9.16 Boxplot and normal probability plot for yields in Example 9.15

9.4 Problems

Problem 9.1. The island of South Georgia is close to the western coast of Antarctica and home to three breeding species of penguins: the king penguin, the gentoo penguin and chinstrap penguin. The following data gives the lengths of 33 penguins measured from the tip of the bill to the tip of the tail, in an outstretched bird:

King	Gentoo	Chinstrap	King	Gentoo	Chinstrap
93.2	78.5	73.2	93.1	80.4	72.5
91.2	79.2	76.3	89.5	77.3	76.3
94.1	81.2	74.5	92.1	78.4	74.9
89.3	83.5	74.9	86.7	82.3	75.2
88.6	79.1	75.2	91.3	80.4	73.7
90.5	81.5	73.1			

(a) Calculate the mean and standard deviation for each group.
(b) Give the median, quartiles and IQR for each group.
(c) Construct the side-by-side box plots for the three groups. What do you observe?
(d) Construct the histograms for the three groups. What do you observe?

Problem 9.2. Redwoods (or sequoias) are the tallest and largest trees on Earth, which can live up to 3,000 years or more. The following table gives the heights and the diameters at breast height (in meters) for a sample of 10 large redwoods in the Redwood National and States Park in Northern California.

Height	Diameter	Height	Diameter
93.57	7.22	80.47	6.16
91.44	6.25	95.71	6.00
97.54	7.92	99.06	6.90
103.94	7.10	65.53	5.79
87.17	7.22	77.72	6.40

(a) Calculate the mean and standard deviation for the heights and for the diameters.
(b) Draw a scatter plot of the heights (x) against the diameters (y).
(c) Calculate the sample covariance and the sample correlation between the heights and the diameters.

Problem 9.3. Sweat bee is a common name for any bee which is attracted to human sweat. The most common species are green or red. The following data gives the color and length (in mm) for 15 sweat bees:

Length	Color	Length	Color	Length	Color
7.5	red	7.3	red	9.1	green
5.6	green	8.2	green	7.3	green
6.7	red	7.3	red	5.6	red
6.9	red	8.6	green	6.6	red
5.4	green	4.8	red	7.5	red

(a) Calculate the mean and median length. Construct the histogram and box plot for the lengths (regardless of the color).
(b) Divide the data into 2 groups consisting of the green bees, respectively the red bees. Calculate the mean and median for each group. Construct the histograms and box plots for each group. What do you observe?

Problem 9.4. The following data gives the blood glucose level (in mmol/L) for 12 persons who suffer from hypoglycemia (low blood glucose levels), before the first meal of the day:

4.2 4.6 4.7 4.5 4.3 4.2 5.1 4.9 4.4 4.6 4.9 5.6

(a) Find the median, and the two quartiles.
(b) Calculate the IQR. Are there any outliers?

Problem 9.5. Henry Cavendish performed a series of experiments in the late 18th century to measure the density of the earth (see [37]). His measurements of the density of the earth are below (source: Table 8 in [52]).

5.50	5.55	5.57	5.34	5.42	5.30
5.61	5.36	5.53	5.79	5.47	5.75
4.88	5.29	5.62	5.10	5.63	5.68
5.07	5.58	5.29	5.27	5.34	5.85
5.26	5.65	5.44	5.39	5.46	

(a) Calculate the mean and median for this data set.
(b) Construct a box plot, a histogram (use 6 bins) and a QQ-plot of the data. Comment on the plots.
(c) Cavendish made changes to his apparatus after the sixth measurement. He considered this change as potentially important. Omit the first six observations from 5.50 to 5.55 and construct a box plot, a histogram (use 6 bins) and a QQ-plot of the remaining data. Does the removal of the first six observations appear to have changed the shape of the distribution?

Problem 9.6. Carbon monoxide is a gas that is highly toxic. The authors of [14] observed that it was possible to have higher mean concentrations of carbon monoxide at urban intersections, compared to highways with much greater traffic volumes. The tables below give the measurements in ppm (parts per million) over a fixed period of time at two different locations.

Location 1

7.6	13.0	8.9	9.4	7.5	8.0	11.2
11.3	10.7	10.9	12.2	11.3	11.9	12.9
11.1	10.4	6.8	9.6	10.3	11.8	11.1
11.3	7.4	8.7	8.5	7.2	7.3	8.4
13.9	10.5	10.6	11.3	11.4	15.6	
11.0	13.8	8.1	10.4	9.1	12.0	

Location 2

10.3	10.6	16.9	7.3	12.3	7.4	16.8
14.0	14.4	19.0	15.4	10.9	13.5	15.4
11.6	16.4	18.9	10.3	15.6	15.2	23.9
16.6	13.7	13.8	11.3	22.2	10.4	6.9
18.3	19.7	16.4	18.6	14.9	14.8	
17.0	16.5	9.4	18.5	14.2	11.3	

(a) Produce side-by-side boxplots for the concentrations of carbon monoxide. Discuss the information that you see in these plots.
(b) Produce overlayed QQ-plots (or normal probability plots) using each sample. Can we compare the variances of the concentration of carbon monoxide variables with these plots? If so, what are your findings?
(c) Does it seem reasonable to assume that the concentration of carbon monoxide is normally distributed?

Problem 9.7. Consider the survival time data from Example 9.6.
(a) Construct a QQ-plot (or a normal probability plot) of the survival times. Does survival time appear to be normally distributed?
(b) Construct a histogram of the survival times. Comment on the shape of the histogram.
(c) Apply a logarithmic transformation to these data. Construct a QQ-plot (or a normal probability plot) of the transformed survival times. Does the transformed survival time appear to be normally distributed?
(d) Construct a histogram of the transformed survival times. Comment on the shape of the histogram.

Problem 9.8. Below we provide the weights of female grizzly bears from two different regions.

Location 1						
191	192	193	197	204	210	218
221	223	229				

Location 2						
159	187	196	200	204	213	219
223	242	249	276	287		

(a) Compute the mean, the standard deviation, the median and the IQR for each group. Are there any outliers?
(b) Construct a histogram for each group and construct side-by-side box plots. Discuss the information that you see in these plots.
(c) Produce QQ-plots for each sample. Do the two weight variables appear to be normally distributed? Discuss how the QQ-plots can be used to compare the variances of the two variables. Are your findings consistent with your discussion from part (b)?

Problem 9.9. We would like to describe the relationship between the mean adult female body mass (in kg) of grizzly bears (y) and the percentage of meat in the diet (x). Below are the data for $n = 12$ different regions.

x	y	x	y
5	120	42	169
6	122	42	171
7	117	60	201
11	129	76	210
12	132	77	225
26	139	79	220

(a) Calculate the mean and standard deviation for the mean adult female body mass and for the percentage of meat in the diet.
(b) Draw a scatter plot of the mean adult female body mass against the percentage of meat in the diet.
(c) Calculate the sample covariance and the sample correlation between the percentage of meat in the diet and the mean adult female body mass.

Chapter 10

Confidence Intervals

In this chapter, we develop a method for estimating an unknown parameter in a certain population. This parameter can be the population mean μ, the population variance σ^2, or the proportion p of individuals with a certain characteristic. As opposed to the method of point estimation, the new method provides a range (or interval) of possible values which contains the unknown parameter with a large probability.

10.1 Confidence Intervals for the Mean: σ^2 Known

In this section, we introduce the method of estimation by confidence intervals for the population mean μ, when the population variance σ^2 is known.

In each of the following examples, we denote by X a random measurement, whose value cannot be predicted with certainty, until the actual measurement is taken. The numerical value of X (that we record when we perform the measurement) is denoted by x. We denote by μ the mean of X, and by σ^2 the variance of X, that is:

$$\mu = E(X), \quad \sigma^2 = \text{Var}(X).$$

By Definition 9.1, a random sample of size n (selected from a population) is a collection of n random measurements, denoted by $X_1, X_2, \ldots, X_n$. These measurements are independent and identically distributed. The observed numerical values (recorded respectively for $X_1, X_2, \ldots, X_n$) are denoted by $x_1, x_2, \ldots, x_n$.

Example 10.1. A research project supported in part by the Canadian Wildlife Federation, shows that in the recent years, an increased number of polar bears in the Beauford Sea are eating less, possibly due to a decrease in the number of ringed seals (the bear's main food source), during a critical spring feeding period. (Additional information about this project can be found in [53]). Further indication that the bears are fasting are smaller weights of their cubs at birth. The following data gives the weights at birth (in grams), for a sample of $n = 5$ cubs:

$$x_1 = 785, \quad x_2 = 825 \quad x_3 = 671 \quad x_4 = 981 \quad x_5 = 732.$$

The average weight for these 5 cubs is:

$$\bar{x} = \frac{785 + 825 + 671 + 981 + 732}{5} = 798.8\text{g}.$$

The sample variance for this data is:

$$s^2 = \frac{1}{5-1}[(785 - 798.8)^2 + (825 - 798.8)^2 + (671 - 798.8)^2 + (981 - 798.8)^2 + (732 - 798.8)^2] = 13717.2.$$

The sample standard deviation is $s = \sqrt{13717.2} = 117.1205\text{g}$. In this example, X represents the weight of a (randomly chosen) cub at birth. We are interested in estimating the mean μ and variance σ^2 of X. From the practical point of view, μ can be interpreted as the average cub weight at birth for the entire population of polar bears in the Beauford Sea, whereas σ gives an indication about the amount of variability of the cub weights at birth. A point estimate for μ is $\bar{x} = 798.8\text{g}$, whereas a point estimate for σ is $s = 117.1205\text{g}$.

Example 10.2. In most cities, the drinking water distributed through the supply network is lead-free. However, it is possible to have traces of lead dissolve into drinking water trough contact with lead service pipes, which were commonly used before 1955. The Health Canada maximum acceptable concentration is 10 ppb (parts per billion). Lead has been identified as a potential human carcinogen. Exposure to low levels of lead over long periods can cause high blood pressure, anaemia, and damage to the peripheral nervous system. The drinking water in 8 houses located in different neighborhoods of Ottawa was tested for lead. For each house, the measurement x represents the lead concentration in drinking water (in ppb).

$$x_1 = 2.1, \quad x_2 = 1.9, \quad x_3 = 2.7, \quad x_4 = 3.1$$

$$x_5 = 5.6, \quad x_6 = 3.3, \quad x_7 = 1.5, \quad x_8 = 0.4.$$

For these 8 houses, the average concentration of lead in drinking water is:

$$\bar{x} = \frac{2.1 + 1.9 + 2.7 + 3.1 + 5.6 + 3.3 + 1.5 + 0.4}{8} = 2.575,$$

which is below the admissible standards. The sample variance is:

$$s^2 = \frac{1}{8-1}\left[(2.1-2.575)^2 + \cdots + (0.4-2.575)^2\right] = 2.362.$$

The sample standard deviation is $s = \sqrt{2.362} = 1.537$. In this example, X represents the lead concentration in drinking water in a (randomly chosen) house in Ottawa. We are interested in estimating the parameter $\mu = E(X)$, which is interpreted as the average concentration of lead in drinking water for the whole city, as well as the parameter $\sigma^2 = \text{Var}(X)$, which gives an indication about the variability of the lead concentration. Point estimates for μ and σ are $\bar{x} = 2.575$, respectively $s = 1.537$.

In the previous examples, $\bar{x}$ is the observed value of the random measurement:

$$\bar{X} = \frac{X_1 + X_2 + \cdots + X_n}{n},$$

whereas s^2 is the observed value of the random measurement:

$$S^2 = \frac{(X_1-\bar{X})^2 + (X_2-\bar{X})^2 + \cdots + (X_n-\bar{X})^2}{n-1}.$$

Both $\bar{X}$ and S^2 are functions of the random sample $X_1, X_2, \ldots, X_n$. They are used for estimating the parameters μ, respectively σ^2. According to Definition 9.2, $\bar{X}$ and S^2 are estimators of μ and σ^2, whereas $\bar{x}$ and s^2 are estimates of μ and σ^2.

Each time a new sample is drawn from the population, the observed (numerical) values $x_1, x_2, \ldots, x_n$ change, but we keep the same notation for the (theoretical) values $X_1, X_2, \ldots, X_n$. One way of keeping track of all the possible (numerical) values $\bar{x}$ and s^2 encountered for different samples, is by examining the probabilistic behavior of the estimators $\bar{X}$ and S^2.

Although the observed value of an estimator cannot be predicted with certainty, when the sample size becomes large, the fluctuation of its possible values becomes less mysterious. In the case of $\bar{X}$, this fluctuation is described by the following statement: (see Theorem 9.5)

$$\frac{\bar{X}-\mu}{\sigma/\sqrt{n}} \quad \text{has approximately a } N(0,1) \text{ distribution,} \qquad (10.1)$$

if n is large enough. Note that if X has a normal distribution with mean μ and variance σ^2, then by Theorem 9.3,

$$\frac{\bar{X}-\mu}{\sigma/\sqrt{n}} \quad \text{has as a } N(0,1) \text{ distribution, for any sample size } n. \qquad (10.2)$$

In this section, we assume that the variance σ^2 is known, and we are interested in estimating μ. Although in most cases this is not a realistic assumption, it helps us understand the general procedure.

Let Z be a random variable with a $N(0,1)$ distribution. We are first interested in finding a point z such that $P(-z \le Z \le z) = 0.95$. This means that $P(Z > z) = (1 - 0.95)/2 = 0.025$ and hence $P(Z \le z) = 1 - 0.025 = 0.975$.

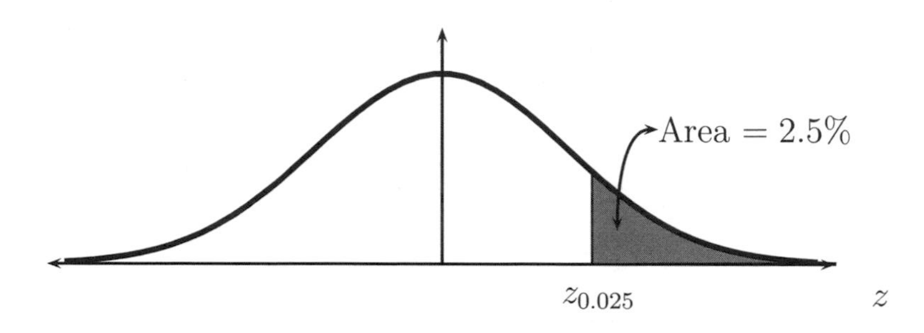

Fig. 10.1 $N(0,1)$ distribution

From Table 17.3, we see that $z = 1.96$, that is:

$$P(-1.96 \le Z \le 1.96) = 0.95.$$

In view of (10.1), we can replace Z by the ratio $(\bar{X} - \mu)/(\sigma/\sqrt{n})$, inferring that:

$$P\left(-1.96 \le \frac{\bar{X} - \mu}{\sigma/\sqrt{n}} \le 1.96\right) = 0.95. \tag{10.3}$$

We now perform a little algebra on the double inequality which characterizes the event above. Note that the inequality

$$\frac{\bar{X} - \mu}{\sigma/\sqrt{n}} \le 1.96$$

is equivalent to $\bar{X} \le \mu + (1.96)(\sigma/\sqrt{n})$, which can be expressed as $\mu \ge \bar{X} - (1.96)(\sigma/\sqrt{n})$. On the other hand, the inequality

$$\frac{\bar{X} - \mu}{\sigma/\sqrt{n}} \ge -1.96$$

tells us that $\bar{X} \ge \mu - (1.96)(\sigma/\sqrt{n})$, which can be expressed as $\mu \le \bar{X} + (1.96)(\sigma/\sqrt{n})$. Therefore, (10.3) becomes

$$P\left(\bar{X} - (1.96)\frac{\sigma}{\sqrt{n}} \le \mu \le \bar{X} + (1.96)\frac{\sigma}{\sqrt{n}}\right) = 0.95. \tag{10.4}$$

Since we assume that the variance σ^2 is known, we conclude that with a probability of 95%, the unknown parameter μ lies between the bounds:

$$L_1 = \bar{X} - (1.96)\frac{\sigma}{\sqrt{n}} \quad \text{and} \quad L_2 = \bar{X} + (1.96)\frac{\sigma}{\sqrt{n}}.$$

Both bounds can be calculated from the observed sample values, since they rely only on $\bar{X}$ and n. In fact, every time we select a new sample, we obtain some new values for L_1 and L_2, leading to a new interval $[L_1, L_2]$. The probability that such a random interval will contain the parameter μ is 95%.

Definition 10.1. The method of **interval estimation** gives a range $[L_1, L_2]$ of values such that the probability that the unknown parameter lies in this range is very large and fixed (typically 95%), and the bounds L_1 and L_2 can be calculated from the sample.

The previous calculation shows that a 95% confidence interval for μ is:

$$\left[\bar{X} - (1.96)\frac{\sigma}{\sqrt{n}},\ \ \bar{X} + (1.96)\frac{\sigma}{\sqrt{n}}\right].$$

Similarly, for deriving the 90% confidence interval for μ, we have to find the point z such that $P(-z \leq Z \leq z) = 0.90$. This means that $P(Z > z) = (1 - 0.90)/2 = 0.05$ and hence $P(Z \leq z) = 1 - 0.5 = 0.95$. From Table 17.3, we find $P(Z < 1.64) = 0.9495$ and $P(Z < 1.65) = 0.9505$. We take z to be the midpoint between 1.64 and 1.65, that is $z = 1.645$. Now, using the fact that

$$P(-1.645 \leq Z \leq 1.645) = 0.90,$$

we conclude that a 90% confidence interval for μ is:

$$\left[\bar{X} - (1.645)\frac{\sigma}{\sqrt{n}},\ \ \bar{X} + (1.645)\frac{\sigma}{\sqrt{n}}\right].$$

To find a 99% confidence interval, we need to find the point z such that $P(-z \leq Z \leq z) = 0.99$. This means that $P(Z > z) = (1 - 0.99)/2 = 0.005$ and hence, $P(Z \leq z) = 1 - 0.005 = 0.995$. Using Table 17.3, we see that $P(Z \leq 2.57) = 0.9949$ and $P(Z \leq 2.58) = 0.9951$. We take $z = 2.575$. Using the same logic as above, and the fact that

$$P(-2.575 \leq Z \leq 2.575) = 0.99,$$

we can show that a 99% confidence interval for μ is:

$$\left[\bar{X} - (2.575)\frac{\sigma}{\sqrt{n}},\ \ \bar{X} + (2.575)\frac{\sigma}{\sqrt{n}}\right].$$

In general, if z is the number that we find using Table 17.3, such that

$$P(-z \leq Z \leq z) = 1 - \alpha$$

then a $100(1-\alpha)\%$ confidence interval for μ is:

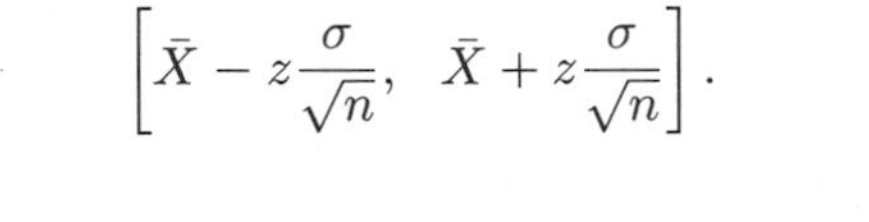

$$\left[\bar{X} - z\frac{\sigma}{\sqrt{n}},\ \bar{X} + z\frac{\sigma}{\sqrt{n}}\right].$$

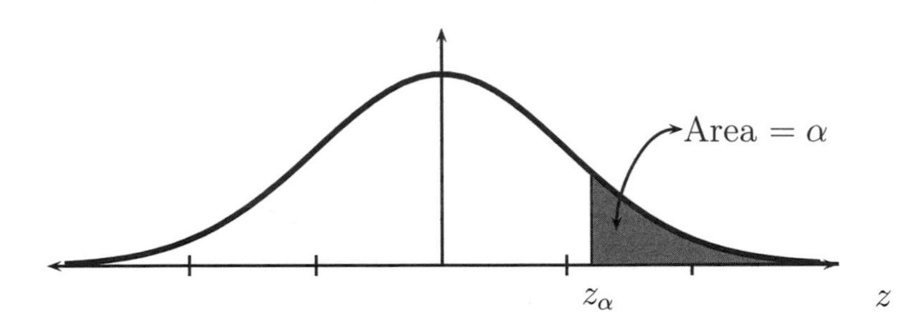

Fig. 10.2 $N(0,1)$ distribution

The interval can be interpreted by saying that we are $100(1-\alpha)\%$ confident that the population average μ lies between $\bar{x} - z(\sigma/\sqrt{n})$ and $\bar{x} + z(\sigma/\sqrt{n})$. Alternatively, we have the following interpretation: if samples are repeatedly drawn from the population, and the confidence interval corresponding to each sample is calculated, we expect that approximately $100(1-\alpha)\%$ of these intervals contain the true mean μ, $100(1-\alpha)\%$ being the confidence level used for calculating the intervals.

Note that, for the same sample size n, the intervals become wider as we increase the probability. Unfortunately, a wide interval is not very useful, despite the fact that it contains the parameter with a large probability. Usually, one would like to balance the negative effect of a too wide interval with the positive fact that it contains the parameter with a large probability. This balance is typically achieved for the 95% confidence intervals.

We also observe that the interval becomes shorter as n becomes larger, since the length of the interval is proportional to $\sigma/\sqrt{n}$.

Example 10.1 (Continued). Suppose that the cub weight X at birth is a normal random variable with standard deviation $\sigma = 115$g. The general formula for the 95% confidence interval is

$$\bar{x} \pm 1.96 \left(\frac{\sigma}{\sqrt{n}} \right).$$

Since X has a normal distribution, the construction of the interval is justified by statement (10.2), even if the sample size is small. We know that $n = 5$, $\bar{x} = 798.8$g and $\sigma = 115$g. A 95% confidence interval for the average cub weight μ at birth is

$$798.8 \pm 1.96 \left(\frac{115}{\sqrt{5}} \right) = 798.8 \pm 100.8 = [698.0;\ 899.6].$$

We are 95% confident that the average cub weight lies between 698.0g and 899.6g.

Suppose now that the cub weight X at birth has a standard deviation $\sigma = 123$g. A new sample of 45 cubs is selected, yielding a sample mean $\bar{x} = 715$g. Even if the distribution of X is not necessarily normal, the sample size is large enough, and the construction of the interval is justified by (10.1). The calculation of the interval is based on $n = 45, \bar{x} = 715$ and $\sigma = 123$. Using this new data, we conclude that a 95% confidence interval for the average cub weight μ at birth is:

$$715 \pm 1.96 \left(\frac{123}{\sqrt{45}} \right) = 715 \pm 35.94 = [679.06;\ 750.94].$$

The interval is shorter than the one found in the first case, mostly because the sample size is larger.

Example 10.2 (Continued). Suppose that the lead concentration X is a normal random variable with standard deviation $\sigma = 1.4$g. We construct a 90% confidence interval for the average lead concentration μ.

The formula for the interval is:

$$\bar{x} \pm 1.645 \left(\frac{\sigma}{\sqrt{n}} \right).$$

The sample size is small, but the measurement X is supposed to be normal. Therefore, the interval calculation is justified by (10.2). We have: $n = 8, \bar{x} = 2.575$ and $\sigma = 1.4$. A 90% interval is:

$$2.575 \pm (1.645) \left(\frac{1.4}{\sqrt{8}} \right) = 2.575 \pm 0.814 = [1.76;\ 3.39].$$

Suppose now that the lead concentration X has a standard deviation $\sigma = 2.6$g. A new sample of 105 houses is selected, yielding a sample mean $\bar{x} = 4.15$g. In this case, the sample size is large, and the interval calculation is justified by (10.1). Suppose that we are interested in finding a 97% confidence interval for the average lead concentration μ at birth, based on this new sample. For this, we have to find a value z such that

$$P(-z \leq Z \leq z) = 0.97.$$

This means that $P(Z > z) = (1 - 0.97)/2 = 0.015$, and therefore $P(Z \leq z) = 1 - 0.015 = 0.985$. From Table 17.3, we see that $z = 2.17$. The formula for the 97% interval is:

$$\bar{x} \pm 2.17 \left(\frac{\sigma}{\sqrt{n}} \right).$$

In our case, $n = 105$, $\bar{x} = 4.15$ and $\sigma = 2.6$. The interval is:

$$4.15 \pm 2.17 \left(\frac{2.6}{\sqrt{105}} \right) = 4.15 \pm 0.55 = [3.6;\ 4.7].$$

We are 97% confident that the average lead concentration μ in drinking water for the city of Ottawa is between 3.6 ppb and 4.7 ppb. If we repeatedly select samples of 105 houses, and we calculate the interval for each of these samples, we expect that 97% of these intervals contain the value μ.

10.2 Confidence Intervals for the Mean: σ^2 Unknown

In Section 10.1, we learned how to build a confidence interval for the unknown mean μ of a population. In order to build this interval, it was essential to know the theoretical value σ^2 of the variance of the population. This is not a realistic assumption since in most cases σ^2 is unknown.

In this section we see how we can circumvent this difficulty, i.e. how we can build a confidence interval for the mean which is based only on numeric values that can be calculated from the sample.

Example 10.3. A study was trying to determine if a drug called "dobutamine" could be used effectively in a test for measuring a patient's risk of having a heart attack, or a "cardiac event". (More details about this study can be found in [23].) For younger patients, a typical test of this risk is called "Stress Echocardiography". It involves raising the patient's heart rate by exercise (often by having the patient run on a treadmill), and then taking various measurements on the heart rate. The measurement X represents the peak heart rate for a patient who is administered this drug. The following data gives the peak heart rate for a sample of 10 patients who participated in this study:

$$x_1 = 130, \quad x_2 = 73, \quad x_3 = 156, \quad x_4 = 123, \quad x_5 = 140$$

$$x_6 = 146, \quad x_7 = 116, \quad x_8 = 136, \quad x_9 = 110, \quad x_{10} = 108.$$

The average peak heart rate for this sample is

$$\bar{x} = \frac{130 + 73 + 156 + 123 + 140 + 146 + 116 + 136 + 110 + 108}{10} = 123.8,$$

and the sample variance is:

$$s^2 = \frac{1}{10-1}\left[(130 - 123.8)^2 + \cdots + (108 - 123.8)^2\right] = 562.4.$$

The sample standard deviation is $s = \sqrt{562.4} = 23.714$. We are interested in estimating the average peak heart rate for patients who are administered this drug.

Example 10.4. The Galápagos archipelago located in the Eastern Pacific Ocean, off Ecuador's coast, is renowned for its rich bio-diversity. Due to its proximity to the Equator, the archipelago has a climate with little variation in daily temperature around the year. During the dry season (June-December), the average daily temperature is between 21^0–23^0C, whereas during the warm season (January-May), the average daily temperature is between 25^0–28^0C. The following data gives the average daily temperature on San Cristóbal island, for 7 days during the dry season:

$$x_1 = 23 \quad x_2 = 20.5, \quad x_3 = 23, \quad x_4 = 19, \quad x_5 = 21, \quad x_6 = 22, \quad x_7 = 22.$$

The average temperature for this sample is

$$\bar{x} = \frac{23 + 20.5 + 23 + 19 + 21 + 22 + 22}{7} = 21.5,$$

and the sample variance is:

$$s^2 = \frac{1}{7-1}\left[(23 - 21.5)^2 + (20.5 - 21.5)^2 + \cdots + (22 - 21.5)^2\right] = 2.083.$$

The sample standard deviation is $s = \sqrt{2.083} = 1.443$. We are interested in estimating the average daily temperature on San Cristóbal island during the dry season.

From Section 9.2, we know that an estimator of the standard deviation σ is the sample standard deviation S.

If we replace σ with its estimator S, then (10.1) fails. However, if we assume that the measurement X has a normal distribution, then the behaviour of the studentized ratio $(\bar{X} - \mu)/(S/\sqrt{n})$ is well-known. More precisely, by Theorem 9.4

$$\frac{\bar{X} - \mu}{S/\sqrt{n}} \quad \text{has a } T(n-1) \text{ distribution.}$$

The confidence interval for μ is constructed using the same technique as in Section 10.1. More precisely, let T be a random variable with a $T(9)$ distribution (which would correspond to a sample of size $n = 10$). From Table 17.4, we know that

$$P(-2.262 \le T \le 2.262) = 0.95.$$

(Note that the area to the right of the point 2.262 is $(1 - 0.95)/2 = 0.025$.) Replacing T by the ratio $(\bar{X} - \mu)/(S/\sqrt{n})$, we infer that:

$$P\left(-2.262 \le \frac{\bar{X} - \mu}{S/\sqrt{n}} \le 2.262\right) = 0.95, \tag{10.5}$$

which can be written as:

$$P\left(\bar{X} - (2.262)\frac{S}{\sqrt{n}} \le \mu \le \bar{X} + (2.262)\frac{S}{\sqrt{n}}\right) = 0.95. \tag{10.6}$$

In conclusion, when X has a normal distribution and we are using a sample of size $n = 10$, a 95% confidence interval for the mean μ is:

$$\left[\bar{X} - (2.262)\frac{S}{\sqrt{n}},\ \bar{X} + (2.262)\frac{S}{\sqrt{n}}\right].$$

Note that the interval bounds can be calculated from the observed sample values (they rely only on $\bar{X}$ and S).

For a general sample size n, if T is a random variable with a $T(n-1)$ distribution, and t is the number found in Table 17.4 such that

$$P(-t \le T \le t) = 1 - \alpha$$

(for a small value α), then a $100(1-\alpha)\%$ confidence interval for μ is:

$$\left[\bar{X} - t\frac{S}{\sqrt{n}},\ \bar{X} + t\frac{S}{\sqrt{n}}\right]. \tag{10.7}$$

Note that in practice, the length of the interval depends on the estimated standard error of the mean $s\{\bar{X}\} = s/\sqrt{n}$.

Example 10.3 (Continued). Assume that the peak heart rate X has a normal distribution, whose variance σ^2 is unknown. We are interested in finding a 95% confidence interval for the average peak heart rate μ.

From the data, we get the estimate $\bar{x} = 123.8$ for the mean μ, the estimate $s = 23.714$ for the standard deviation σ, and the estimate $s^2 = 562.4$ for the variance σ^2. These are all point estimators.

In this case, the confidence interval is based on a random variable T with a $T(9)$ distribution. For the 95% level of confidence, we use $t = 2.262$. Therefore, a 95% confidence interval for μ is

$$123.8 \pm 2.262\left(\frac{23.714}{\sqrt{10}}\right) = 123.8 \pm 16.96 = [106.84;\ 140.76].$$

Suppose that for a new sample of 25 patients, the sample mean is $\bar{x} = 115.0$ and the sample variance is $s^2 = 643.5$. We want to find a 90% confidence interval for μ.

This confidence interval is based on a random variable T with a $T(24)$ distribution. For the 90% level of confidence, we have to find a value t such that $P(-t \leq T \leq t) = 0.90$. Then $P(T \geq t) = (1 - 0.90)/2 = 0.05$ and hence $P(T \leq t) = 1 - 0.05 = 0.95$. Table 17.4 gives the value $t = 1.711$. Therefore, a 90% confidence interval for μ is

$$115.0 \pm 1.711 \left(\frac{\sqrt{643.5}}{\sqrt{25}} \right) = 115.0 \pm 8.68 = [106.32;\ 123.68].$$

Example 10.4 (Continued). Assume that the daily temperature X (during the dry season) has a normal distribution. We want to find a 90% confidence interval for the average average daily temperature μ during the dry season.

We have $\bar{x} = 21.5$ and $s^2 = 2.083$. The confidence interval is based on a random variable T with a $T(6)$ distribution. To construct the interval, we have first to find the value t such that $P(-t \leq T \leq t) = 0.90$, where T is a random variable with a $T(6)$ distribution. This means that $P(T > t) = (1 - 0.90)/2 = 0.05$ and $P(T \leq t) = 1 - 0.05 = 0.95$. From Table 17.4, we find $t = 1.943$. A 90% confidence interval for μ is

$$21.5 \pm 1.943 \left(\frac{\sqrt{2.083}}{\sqrt{7}} \right) = 21.5 \pm 1.06 = [20.44;\ 22.56].$$

We should point out that in practice, if the sample size is large (i.e. $n \geq 40$), one may replace the value t in (10.7) with the value z, such that $P(-z \leq Z \leq z) = 1 - \alpha$. This is called a *large sample interval*, and is justified by the fact that the distribution of the studentized sample mean becomes approximately standard normal, as the sample size becomes very large (see Theorem 9.5).

10.3 Confidence Intervals for the Proportion

In this section, we discuss the method of estimation by confidence intervals, when the parameter of interest is the proportion p of individuals who possess a certain characteristic. In probabilistic terms, p is the proportion of "successes" in a given population. For example, p can be the proportion of voters favorable to a certain political candidate, the proportion of people affected by a disease, or the proportion of patients who suffer from side-effects due to a medication.

Suppose that a random sample of n individuals is selected from the population, and this sample contains Y individuals who possess the characteristic. Note that Y is a random measurement, since it depends on the random sample: each time we select a new sample, the value of Y changes. Let p be the proportion of individuals from the population who possess the characteristic, and suppose that p is unknown. An estimator for p is:

$$\hat{p} = \frac{Y}{n}.$$

Note that the estimator $\hat{p}$ coincides with a particular instance of the estimator $\bar{X}$. To see this, we associate to each individual in the sample, a measurement X which takes only the values 0 or 1. More precisely, for the i-th individual in the sample, we define the random measurement:

$$X_i = \begin{cases} 1 \text{ if the individual } i \text{ is a "success} \\ 0 \text{ if the individual } i \text{ is a "failure".} \end{cases}$$

Since $\sum_{i=1}^{n} X_i = Y$, the mean of the sample $X_1, \ldots, X_n$ is:

$$\bar{X} = \frac{1}{n} \sum_{i=1}^{n} X_i = \frac{1}{n} Y = \hat{p}.$$

Therefore, the estimation procedure that we develop in the present section is a particular case of the method developed in Section 10.1.

Example 10.5. During an election campaign, we are interested in estimating the percentage of voters who are in favor of a certain political candidate. In a sample of $n = 300$ randomly selected voters, there are $y = 21$ who are in favor of the candidate. The estimate for the (unknown) proportion p of voters who are in favor of the candidate is:

$$\hat{p} = \frac{21}{300} = 0.07, \quad \text{or} \quad 7\%.$$

Example 10.6. A physician is interested in estimating the proportion p of patients treated with a certain drug, who suffer undesirable side effects. In a sample of $n = 200$ patients, $y = 5$ patients suffered side effects. An estimate for p is:

$$\hat{p} = \frac{5}{200} = 0.025, \quad \text{or} \quad 2.5\%.$$

Example 10.7. According to an article in the National Geographic magazine (September 2007), the gene responsible for human's red hair is thought to be due to a mutation, which took place in northern Europe thousands of years ago. It is estimated that the red hair people will become extinct by the year 2100, since the gene is recessive and the percentage of people carrying it around the world is very low (around 4%). The country with the largest percentage of red hair people is Scotland. In a sample of 2,500 Scots, 325 have red hair. Based on this data, an estimate for the percentage p of Scotland's population who has red hair is:

$$\hat{p} = \frac{325}{2,500} = 0.13, \quad \text{or} \quad 13\%.$$

Example 10.8. One of the difficulties encountered when trying to fight AIDS is that the number of people infected with HIV around the world is unknown. According to a 2007 United Nations report on AIDS epidemic, South Africa is the country with the largest number of HIV infections in the world. In a sample of 8,500 South Africans, 935 were infected with the HIV. Based on this data, the proportion of the South Africa's population infected with the HIV is:

$$\hat{p} = \frac{935}{8,500} = 0.11, \quad \text{or} \quad 11\%.$$

To build a confidence interval for the proportion p of "successes" in a population, we need to have a better understanding of the fluctuations of $\hat{p}$. Such understanding is provided by the following statement, which is a particular instance of (10.1):

$$\frac{\hat{p} - p}{\sqrt{p(1-p)/n}} \quad \text{has approximately a } N(0,1) \text{ distribution,} \quad \text{if } n \text{ is large.}$$

If the sample size is very large (i.e. larger than 100), one can replace the unknown value $p(1-p)$ under the square root above, by its estimator $\hat{p}(1-\hat{p})$, without destroying the $N(0,1)$ distribution. More precisely,

$$\frac{\hat{p} - p}{\sqrt{\hat{p}(1-\hat{p})/n}} \quad \text{has approximately a } N(0,1) \text{ distribution,} \tag{10.8}$$

if n is very large. Recall that if Z is a random variable with a $N(0,1)$ distribution, then

$$P(-1.96 \leq Z \leq 1.96) = 0.95.$$

In view of (10.8), we can replace Z by the ratio $(\hat{p} - p)/\sqrt{\hat{p}(1-\hat{p})/n}$, inferring that:

$$P\left(-1.96 \leq \frac{\hat{p} - p}{\sqrt{\hat{p}(1-\hat{p})/n}} \leq 1.96\right) = 0.95, \tag{10.9}$$

which can be written as:

$$P\left(\hat{p} - (1.96)\sqrt{\frac{\hat{p}(1-\hat{p})}{n}} \leq p \leq \hat{p} + (1.96)\sqrt{\frac{\hat{p}(1-\hat{p})}{n}}\right) = 0.95. \tag{10.10}$$

We conclude that with a probability of 95%, the unknown parameter p lies in the interval:

$$\left[\hat{p} - (1.96)\sqrt{\frac{\hat{p}(1-\hat{p})}{n}};\ \hat{p} + (1.96)\sqrt{\frac{\hat{p}(1-\hat{p})}{n}}\right]. \tag{10.11}$$

This is a 95% confidence interval for p, since the interval bounds can be calculated from the data.

Using a similar argument, we infer that the general $100(1-\alpha)\%$-confidence interval for p is:

$$\hat{p} \pm z\sqrt{\frac{\hat{p}(1-\hat{p})}{n}},$$

where z is chosen from Table 17.3 such that $P(-z \leq Z \leq z) = 1 - \alpha$.

Example 10.5 (Continued). We are interested in finding a 95% confidence interval for the proportion p of voters who are in favor of the candidate. Using formula (10.11), the interval is:

$$0.07 \pm 1.96\sqrt{\frac{(0.07)\cdot(0.93)}{300}} = 0.07 \pm 0.029 = [0.041;\ 0.099].$$

We are 95% confident that p is between 4.1% and 9.9%. Alternatively, the result could be interpreted as follows: if samples of 300 voters are repeatedly selected and the interval corresponding to each sample is calculated, then 95% of these intervals contain the proportion p of voters who are in favor of the candidate. The interval is reported in the news as follows: the proportion of voters who are in favor of the candidate is 7%, with a margin of error of 2.9%, the result being valid 19 times out of 20.

Example 10.6 (Continued). A 90% confidence interval for the proportion p of patients who suffer side effects due to the medication is:

$$0.025 \pm 1.645\sqrt{\frac{(0.025)\cdot(0.975)}{200}} = 0.025 \pm 0.018 = [0.007;\ 0.043].$$

The interpretation could be interpreted as follows: if samples of 200 patients are repeatedly used for testing this drug, and the interval corresponding to each sample is calculated, then 90% of these intervals contain the proportion p of patients who suffer side effects.

Example 10.7 (Continued). We are interested in finding a 98% confidence interval for the proportion p of red haired people of Scotland.

We first have to find the point z such that $P(-z \leq Z \leq z) = 0.98$. This means that $P(Z > z) = (1-0.98)/2 = 0.01$ and $P(Z \leq z) = 1-0.1 = 0.99$. From Table 17.3, we find $z = 2.33$. A 98% confidence interval is:

$$0.13 \pm 2.33\sqrt{\frac{(0.13)\cdot(0.87)}{2,500}} = 0.13 \pm 0.016 = [0.114;\ 0.146].$$

We are 98% confident that p is between 11.4% and 14.6%.

Example 10.8 (Continued). According to formula (10.11), a 95% confidence interval for the proportion p of HIV infected people in South Africa in 2007 is:

$$0.11 \pm 1.96\sqrt{\frac{(0.11)\cdot(0.89)}{8,500}} = 0.11 \pm 0.0067 = [0.1033;\ 0.1167].$$

We are 95% confident that p is between 10.33% and 11.67%.

It is known that the population of South Africa was 47.9 million in 2007. Using this information, we can give a 95% confidence interval for the number of HIV infected people in South Africa in 2007. The lower bound for the estimated number of HIV infected people is $(47.9)(0.1033) = 4.95$ million. The upper bound is $(47.9)(0.1167) = 5.59$ million. In conclusion, we are 95% confident that the number of people who were infected with HIV in South Africa in 2007 is between 4.95 million and 5.59 million.

10.4 Problems

Problem 10.1. One of the high risk HIV groups are injecting drug users (IUDs). In a group of 1,000 IUD's, it was reported that 186 of them were infected with HIV. Find a point estimate and a 90% confidence interval for the proportion p of HIV carriers in the IUD population.

Problem 10.2. In the recent years, there was an increase in the percentage of the population who favors the medical use of marijuana for patients suffering from severe illnesses (for instance, to help cancer patients deal with chemotherapy). In the United States, the laws on medical use of marijuana are being tested on a state-by-state basis. According to [45], a 2002 survey of 600 residents of Wisconsin, conducted by Chamberlain Research Consultants found that 480 favored a law that would allow seriously ill or terminally ill patients to use marijuana for medical purposes, if supported by their physician. Give a 95% confidence interval for the proportion of the Wisconsin population in favor of the medical use of marijuana. Interpret the result.

Problem 10.3. Platelet monoamine oxidase (MAO) is an index of brain serotonin activity. Low MAO levels have been found to be related to behavior disorders. In the study [15], the MAO activity levels of 30 patients with bulimia nervosa were measured. The average level of MAO activity for the 30 bulimic patients was 4.4 nmol/10^8 platelets/hour, with a standard deviation of 2.4 nmol/10^8 platelets/hour.
(a) Based on this data, give a 95% confidence interval for the average MAO activity level of bulimic patients. Assume that the level of MAO activity is normally distributed.
(b) The normal range for the MAO levels is between 5.5 and 8.5. How does the interval constructed in part (a) compare with the normal range? What conclusion can be drawn?

Problem 10.4. The following data gives the weight for 8 corn cobs which were produced using an organic corn fertilizer:

212 234 259 189 245 176 203 215

Assume that the cob weight has a normal distribution with standard deviation $\sigma = 28$g. Find a 96% confidence interval for the average cob weight. Interpret the result.

Problem 10.5. Water hardness is a traditional measure of the capacity of water to react with soap. Hardness in water is caused by dissolved calcium and magnesium. It is expressed as the equivalent quantity of calcium carbonate (see [57]). Fifteen measurements were collected from randomly chosen lakes in a particular district. The mean hardness is 102.03 mg/l and the estimated standard error of the mean is 1.378 mg/l.
(a) Give the sample standard deviation of the 15 hardness measurements.
(b) Assuming that water hardness is normally distributed, compute a 95% confidence interval for the mean water hardness.

(c) According to Health Canada (source: www.hc-sc.gc.ca), water with a hardness smaller than 100 mg/l is classified as soft and water with a hardness larger than 180 mg/l is classified as hard. If the hardness is between soft and hard, we say that the water is medium hard. With a level of confidence of 95%, can we classify the mean hardness of the water in this district as medium hard?

Problem 10.6. A farmer has observed that for a certain variety of tomato, a plant will yield on average 2.7 kg of fruit per year. Some soil has been treated with a soil conditioner to increase the yield. Twenty plants in the treated soil had a mean yield of $\overline{x} = 3.1$ kg (per year) and a standard deviation of $s = 0.53$ kg. It was verified that the yield of a plant is normally distributed.
(a) Give a 95% confidence interval for the mean yield of a tomato plant under the new conditions.
(b) Compare the interval estimate from part (a) with the old mean yield. What can we conclude?

Problem 10.7. pH is the negative logarithm of the hydrogen ion activity. It is a measure of how acid or alkaline a substance is on a scale of 0 to 14. A pH of 7 is neutral, less than 7 is acidic and greater than 7 is alkaline. The ideal pH for soil depends on the crop being grown. Levels between 6.5 and 7 are considered optimal for many plants (see [39]). Eighteen samples of soil are randomly selected from a field and are sent to a laboratory for pH measurements. Below are the data.

6.11	6.26	5.67	5.76	7.30	5.68	6.57	6.57	6.07
5.76	5.91	6.16	7.02	6.35	6.77	6.65	7.05	6.85

(a) Produce a normal probability plot for this sample. Do the measurements of pH appear to be normally distributed?
(b) Compute a 95% confidence interval for the mean pH level.

Problem 10.8. A new drug is being tested for its effectiveness to treat a certain type of infection. It was effective in 119 cases out of 170.
(a) Construct a 95% confidence interval for the rate of effectiveness of the new drug for treating this type of infection.
(b) Without constructing the 98% confidence interval for the rate of effectiveness, would you expect the interval to be longer or shorter compared to the 95% confidence interval? Why?

(c) Construct a 98% confidence interval for the rate of effectiveness of the new drug for treating this type of infection.

Did you know that? *Many of the species of the Galápagos archipelago were discovered for the first time by Charles Darwin during his historical voyage around the South American coast, aboard the ship* Beagle *(1831-1836). This expedition is one of the best known episodes in the history of science. As the ship's naturalist, Darwin (then a 22-year old Cambridge graduate) visited the archipelago and was amazed by the curious creatures he encountered (e.g. giant tortoises, finches). It is thought that Darwin's theory of evolution based on natural selection may have its origins in this voyage. (For more details about Darwin's voyage to the Galápagos islands, see* [48]*.)*

Chapter 11

Hypothesis Testing

In this chapter, we introduce another statistical method for drawing conclusions about the values of a parameter. This method consists in confronting two hypotheses which speak about the parameter values. It is used when one wants to gain support (or evidence) towards a desired statement, called "the research hypothesis", and denoted by H_1. The other hypothesis, which the researcher wants to reject, is called the "null hypothesis", and is denoted by H_0. When using this method, we formulate the two hypotheses with the goal of rejecting H_0, and gaining evidence towards H_1.

11.1 Hypothesis Testing for the Mean: σ^2 Known

In this section, we introduce the method of hypothesis testing, when the parameter of interest is the population mean μ, and the population variance σ^2 is known. The null hypothesis H_0 says that the unknown parameter μ is equal to a specified numerical value μ_0:

$$H_0 : \mu = \mu_0.$$

Under new experimental conditions, the mean measurement μ is thought to deviate from μ_0, which is a value obtained under standard conditions. The alternative hypothesis H_1 (that we would like to gain evidence for) specifies the direction of this change in μ. This hypothesis can take three different forms:

(1) μ is larger than μ_0. In this case, we write $H_1 : \mu > \mu_0$, and we say that we perform a *right-tailed test.* This set-up is used when one wants to gain evidence that μ exceeds the hypothesized value μ_0.

(2) μ is smaller than μ_0. In this case, we write $H_1 : \mu < \mu_0$ and we say that we perform a *left-tailed test.* This set-up is used when one wants to gain evidence that μ diminishes compared to μ_0.

(3) μ is different than μ_0. In this case, we write $H_1 : \mu \neq \mu_0$ and we say that we perform a *two-tailed test.* This set-up is used when the direction of the change in μ is unknown.

Setting up the hypothesis in the desired way (i.e. choosing the appropriate alternative hypothesis H_1, among the three possibilities listed above) is the first and most important step of a statistical testing procedure. Before performing the test, the statistician has to decide what is the alternative hypothesis H_1. This decision dictates automatically which of the three cases above has to be used for the problem at hand.

The conclusion of a test of hypothesis is one of the following:

(i) We reject H_0. In this case, we say that there is enough evidence in favor of H_1. (We may say that H_1 is true.)

(ii) We fail to reject H_0. In this case, we say that there is not enough evidence in favor of H_1. (We avoid saying that H_0 is true, although this may help with the logic.)

As a consequence, hypothesis testing can result in two types of errors:

- *Type I error* (whose probability is denoted by α) is encountered if we reject H_0, when H_0 is true.
- *Type II error* (whose probability is denoted by β) is encountered if we fail to reject H_0, when H_1 is true.

Ideally, both probabilities α and β should be small. The table below illustrates all 4 possibilities:

	Reject H_0	Fail to reject H_0
H_0 true	Type I error (probability α)	Correct decision (probability $1 - \alpha$)
H_1 true	Correct decision (probability $1 - \beta$)	Type II error (probability β)

Fig. 11.1 Probabilities associated with a test of hypothesis

Example 11.1. The effects of inhaling particle matter (PM) have been widely studied in humans. The smaller particles PM_{10} (particles with diameter of less that 10 micrometers) are especially dangerous, and possibly related to asthma and lung cancer. As of January 1, 2005 the European Commission has set the limit for the PM_{10} in the air at 50 $\mu g/m^3$ (daily average). Local health organizations in a large European city are concerned that the PM_{10} level in the outdoor air is higher than the 50 $\mu g/m^3$ permissible. To test the validity of this statement, levels of PM_{10} were measured on 25 different days, yielding an average $\bar{x} = 53.5$ $\mu g/m^3$.

To set-up correctly the two hypotheses, we keep in mind that we want to reject H_0, in favor of H_1. Therefore, we set H_0: "the average level of PM_{10} is equal to 50" and H_1: "the average level of PM_{10} exceeds 50". We are confronting the following two hypotheses:

$$H_0 : \mu = 50 \quad \text{versus} \quad H_1 : \mu > 50.$$

A type I error occurs when we decide that the PM_{10} level is higher than 50, when in fact it is not. This does not have a negative health impact, but may result in falsely alarming the public.

A type II error occurs when we are unable to gain evidence that the PM_{10} level is higher than 50, when in fact it is. This may have a negative health effect on the population.

Example 11.2. Cholesterol is one of the body's fats, used for making cell membranes, vitamin D and hormones. High levels of low-density lipoprotein (LDL) cholesterol in the blood can cause the build up of plaque in the artery walls, which is a major risk factor for heart disease and stroke. The Canadian Heart and Stroke Foundation advises a diet low in saturated fats and regular physical activities as effective measures for reducing the LDL blood cholesterol levels. To gain evidence for this statement, we use a sample of 52 Canadians with a high level of LDL blood cholesterol of 4.0 nmol/L, who were on a low-fat diet for 30 days, combined with 30 minutes of daily cardio exercises. After this period, the average LDL blood cholesterol level for this sample was found to be $\bar{x} = 3.5$, which is lower than the initial value $\mu_0 = 4.0$.

We now set-up the two hypotheses in the desired direction. The goal is to reject H_0, and gain evidence for H_1. The null hypothesis $H_0 : \mu = 4.0$ says that despite the new measures, the average LDL blood cholesterol level stays the same. The alternative hypothesis $H_1 : \mu < 4.0$ says that the LDL blood cholesterol level is reduced. We are confronting the following two hypotheses:

$$H_0 : \mu = 4.0 \quad \text{versus} \quad H_1 : \mu < 4.0.$$

A type I error occurs when we decide that diet combined with exercise reduces the LDL blood cholesterol level, when in fact it does not. A type II error occurs if we are unable to gain evidence that diet combined with exercise reduces the LDL blood cholesterol level, when in fact it does.

Example 11.3. Recent studies suggest that Bacillus Calmette-Guérin (BCG) vaccination early in life is related to asthma. A commonly used index of asthma in a population is the level of forced expiratory volume in one second (FEV_1). The level of FEV_1 was measured in 36 adult men, who were administered the BCG vaccine at the age of 14, yielding an average volume $\bar{x} = 4.52$ BTPS. We would like to gain evidence for the fact that the BCG vaccination induces a change in the FEV_1 level, the direction of the change being unknown. For adult men, the normal level of FEV_1 is around the value of 4.00 BTPS.

We set-up the two hypotheses, with the goal of rejecting H_0, in favor of H_1. Hypothesis H_0 says that the BCG vaccination does not induce a significant change in the FEV_1 level. The alternative hypothesis H_1 says that the BCG induces either an increase or a decrease in the FEV_1 level. We want to test:

$$H_0 : \mu = 4.00 \quad \text{versus} \quad H_1 : \mu \neq 4.00,$$

μ being the average FEV_1 level in the BCG-vaccinated male population.

A type I error occurs when we decide that the BCG vaccination induces a change in the FEV_1 level, when in fact it does not. A type II error occurs if we are unable to gain evidence that the BCG vaccination affects the FEV_1 level, when in fact it does.

We treat separately the three different cases, explaining what method to use in each case.

Case (1). $H_0 : \mu = \mu_0$ versus $H_1 : \mu > \mu_0$

This is the case when we want to gain evidence that the true mean μ of the population is larger than a numerical value μ_0. To move in the direction of H_1, we first have to make sure that in the case of our sample, the sample average $\bar{x}$ is larger than μ_0. (If this is not the case, there is no hope that we can gather any evidence for H_1.)

We then calculate the difference $\bar{x} - \mu_0$, and hope that this difference is a large (positive) number. If so, then we reject H_0; otherwise, we say that we do not have enough evidence for rejecting H_0.

But how large should this number be? To answer this question, the difference $\bar{x} - \mu_0$ itself is not of big help. We have to calculate the standardized ratio $z_0 = (\bar{x} - \mu_0)/(\sigma/\sqrt{n})$ and see if this ratio is large, compared with all the possible values for the same ratio that may arise from other samples. The collection of all the samples is huge and therefore, it is impossible to calculate all the corresponding ratios. Luckily, the way these ratios fluctuate is well-known: if H_0 is true, then by Theorem 9.5,

$$Z_0 = \frac{\bar{X} - \mu_0}{\sigma/\sqrt{n}} \quad \text{has approximately a } N(0,1) \text{ distribution,}$$

if n is large enough. (Recall that, if the sample is drawn from a normal population, then the previous statement continues to hold true for any n, and the word "approximately" is replaced by "exactly"; see Theorem 9.3.) In this context, Z_0 is called the *test statistic*.

The question is: supposing that H_0 is true, do we expect to see only rarely sample averages larger than our observed $\bar{x}$, or our $\bar{x}$ is a rather typical value, and we should expect to see very often values which are even larger?

To answer this question, we use Table 17.3 for calculating the probability that a $N(0,1)$ random variable takes a value larger (i.e more extreme) than the value z_0 that we already observed. This probability is called the *p-value of the right-tailed test*:

$$p\text{-value} = P(Z > z_0),$$

and corresponds to the right tail of the $N(0,1)$ density. We say that z_0 is the *observed value of the test statistic* Z_0.

The smaller the p-value, the less likely it is that H_0 is true. The interpretation is the following: a small p-value means that values larger than $\bar{x}$ are rarely encountered under H_0, and therefore H_0 is unlikely to be true. On the other hand, a large p-value means that values larger than $\bar{x}$ are frequently encountered under H_0, and therefore H_0 is likely to be true.

Reporting the p-value is an important step in any statistical analysis, since it gives us an idea about the likelihood that H_0 happens.

Sometimes, statisticians are supplied with an a priori α-value for the probability of the type I error. In this case, the decision rule of the test is based on the following comparison between the p-value and α:

$$\begin{aligned} &\text{if } p\text{-value} < \alpha, \text{ then we reject } H_0 \\ &\text{if } p\text{-value} > \alpha, \text{ then we fail to reject } H_0. \end{aligned}$$

Note that there is some uncertainty in this decision-making process. In fact, a statistician in never 100% sure of making the right decision. The above rule ensures that the probability of the type I error is equal to α.

Example 11.1 (Continued). Suppose that the daily level X of PM_{10} in the city's outdoor air is a normal random variable of unknown mean μ and known variance $\sigma^2 = 33.5$. The sample size is $n = 25$. The sample average $\bar{x} = 53.5$ indicates that the unknown average μ may be higher that the threshold value $\mu_0 = 50$. To gain evidence for this claim, we calculate the ratio:

$$z_0 = \frac{\bar{x} - \mu_0}{\sigma/\sqrt{n}} = \frac{53.5 - 50}{\sqrt{33.5}/\sqrt{25}} = 3.02.$$

We cannot say if the value of this ratio is large or small, until we compare it with all the other possible values, which may arise if we change the sample. This comparison is performed using the p-value. From Table 17.3,

$$p\text{-value} = P(Z > 3.02) = 1 - 0.9987 = 0.0013.$$

This p-value is very small. Based on this sample, it is unlikely that $H_0 : \mu = 50$ is true, and is much more likely that $H_1 : \mu > 50$ is true. Therefore, we have enough evidence for rejecting H_0. The conclusion is that in this city, the average PM_{10} in the outdoor air exceeds the permissible level of 50 $\mu g/m^3$ per day.

Case (2). $H_0 : \mu = \mu_0$ versus $H_1 : \mu < \mu_0$

In this case, we want to gain evidence that the average μ is smaller than a given value μ_0. This time, we first have to make sure that the sample average $\bar{x}$ is smaller than μ_0. Then, we calculate the same ratio $z_0 = (\bar{x} - \mu_0)/(\sigma/\sqrt{n})$, keeping in mind that this (negative) ratio value should be compared against all the other negative values in Table 17.2, which could be obtained from different samples. The p-value is a measure of how "negative" this ratio is compared with all the other values. It gives the probability that one can obtain something even more "negative" (or more extreme) in the case of another sample:

$$p\text{-value} = P(Z < z_0).$$

Note that this probability corresponds to the left-tail of the $N(0,1)$ density. A small p-value means that $\bar{x}$ is sufficiently small compared to μ_0. In this case, we reject H_0, and conclude that there is enough evidence that μ is smaller that μ_0.

As in Case (1), if a preset α-value is given for the probability of the type I error, we reject H_0 if and only if the p-value is smaller than α.

Example 11.2 (Continued). Let X be the LDL blood cholesterol level of a randomly chosen person who was on a low-fat diet for 30 days, combined with daily exercising. Suppose that X has a standard deviation $\sigma = 1.12$. The sample average $\bar{x} = 3.5$ is smaller than the initial cholesterol level of 4.0, so we can proceed with the test. We calculate the ratio:

$$z_0 = \frac{\bar{x} - \mu_0}{\sigma/\sqrt{n}} = \frac{3.5 - 4.0}{1.12/\sqrt{52}} = -3.22.$$

This value is very extreme for the observed value of a Z random variable. More precisely, from Table 17.2,

$$p\text{-value} = P(Z < -3.22) = 0.0006.$$

This is a very small probability. We reject H_0, in favor of H_1. The conclusion of this study is that a low-fat diet and exercising are effective means of reducing the LDL blood cholesterol level.

Case (3). $H_0 : \mu = \mu_0$ versus $H_1 : \mu \neq \mu_0$

In this case, we want to show that the unknown average μ is significantly different than a value μ_0, without any preference for the direction of the change in μ compared to μ_0. This type of test can be performed if $\bar{x}$ is either larger, or smaller than μ_0. What matters is the absolute value of the difference $\bar{x} - \mu_0$. In fact, our conclusion is based on the absolute value of the ratio $z_0 = (\bar{x} - \mu_0)/(\sigma/\sqrt{n})$. If this value is very large (or extreme), then we reject H_0; otherwise, we do not have enough evidence for rejecting H_0.

The p-value calculation takes into account the fact that the same absolute value $|z_0|$ can be encountered in two different situations: when $\bar{x}$ is larger than μ_0, or $\bar{x}$ is smaller than μ_0. Before selecting the sample, we do not know which of these two situations will be encountered in the case of our sample. For this reason, the p-value calculation considers both tails under the $N(0,1)$ density:

$$p\text{-value} = 2P(Z > |z_0|).$$

The value 2 in the formula above is due to the symmetry of the density of the $N(0,1)$ distribution.

As in the previous two cases, we reject H_0 if the p-value is small. Otherwise, we do not have enough evidence for rejecting H_0. If an a priori α-value is given, we reject H_0 if and only if the p-value is smaller than α.

Example 11.3 (Continued). Let X be the FEV_1 level in the BCG-vaccinated male population. We assume that X has a normal distribution with known variance $\sigma^2 = 2.1$. We first calculate the absolute value:

$$|z_0| = \left|\frac{\bar{x} - \mu_0}{\sigma/\sqrt{n}}\right| = \left|\frac{4.52 - 4.00}{\sqrt{2.1}/\sqrt{36}}\right| = 2.15.$$

From Table 17.3, we find

$$p\text{-value} = 2P(Z > 2.15) = 2(1 - 0.9842) = 2(0.0158) = 0.0316.$$

If the preset α-value is given as $\alpha = 0.01$ (i.e. we are willing to accept only a risk of 1% of making a type I error), then we fail to reject H_0, and conclude that there is not enough evidence that the BCG vaccination affects the FEV_1 level. However, if the preset α-value is $\alpha = 0.05$ (i.e. we are willing to accept a risk of 5% of making a type I error), then we reject H_0, and conclude that the BCG vaccination may affect the FEV_1 level.

11.2 Hypothesis Testing for the Mean: σ^2 Unknown

In this section, we modify slightly the procedure developed in the previous section for performing a test on the population average μ, in the case when the population variance σ^2 is unknown, and the measurement X is normally distributed.

We consider separately the three cases:

Case (1). $H_0 : \mu = \mu_0$ versus $H_1 : \mu > \mu_0$

The method is very similar to the one encountered in Section 11.1. A large value of $\bar{x}$ (compared to μ_0) is an indication that H_0 is not true. The only difference is that now it is no longer practical to use the (approximate) normal distribution of the ratio $(\bar{X} - \mu_0)/(\sigma/\sqrt{n})$, since this ratio depends on the unknown quantity σ.

To circumvent this difficulty, we use the same idea as in Section 10.2, replacing σ by its estimate s (the sample standard deviation) and the standard normal distribution $N(0, 1)$ by the $T(n - 1)$ distribution. More precisely, we use the following fact: if H_0 is true, then by Theorem 9.4

$$T_0 = \frac{\bar{X} - \mu_0}{S/\sqrt{n}} \text{ has a } T(n-1) \text{ distribution.}$$

The test is based on the calculation of the studentized ratio $t_0 = (\bar{x} - \mu_0)/(s/\sqrt{n})$. In this case, t_0 is the observed value of the test statistic T_0. A large (positive) value of this ratio is an indication that H_0 is not true. To see if this ratio is really large (compared with other values encountered from different samples), we consider the following:

$$p\text{-value} = P(T > t_0),$$

where T is a random variable with a $T(n-1)$ distribution.

A small p-value is an indication that $\bar{x}$ is sufficiently large. In this case, we reject H_0; otherwise, we fail to reject H_0. If a preset α-value is given, we reject H_0 if and only if the p-value is smaller than α.

We should say few words about the p-value calculation in this case. Due to the limitations of Table 17.4, which gives only the values t corresponding to a selected number of probabilities $P(T \leq t)$, in the examples below we content ourselves with reporting only the interval where the p-value lies. For this, we have to place the ratio t_0 between some values that we identify in Table 17.4, on row $\nu = n - 1$. In some examples, this means finding two values $t_1 < t_2$ (whose corresponding areas to the right are $\alpha_1 > \alpha_2$), such that:

$$t_1 < t_0 < t_2.$$

In this case, we report that:

$$\alpha_2 < p\text{-value} < \alpha_1.$$

In other examples, we may find only one value t_1 (whose corresponding area to the right is α_1), such that:

$$t_0 > t_1.$$

In this case, we report that: p-value $< \alpha_1$. Note that, due to the limitations of this procedure, a comparison with a preset α-value is not always possible. In practice, the exact p-value is obtained using a statistical software.

Example 11.4. Leatherbacks are one of the biggest and deepest living of all sea turtles. Their immense mass of up to 2,000 pounds helps them stay warm in the frigid water. In the recent years, the number and the size of leatherbacks in the Atlantic has increased, due to the abundant jellyfish population off the coasts of Nova Scotia, where they come to feed after nesting on the beaches of Trinidad. The claim is that the average mass of an Atlantic leatherback is now higher that 1,000 pounds. We want to test this claim, using the hypothesis

$$H_0 : \mu = 1,000 \quad \text{versus} \quad H_1 : \mu > 1,000,$$

where μ is the average mass of an Atlantic leatherback.

Type I error occurs when we decide that the average mass of an Atlantic leatherback is higher than 1,000 pounds, when in fact it is not. Type II error occurs if we conclude that there is not enough evidence that the average mass is higher than 1,000 pounds, when in fact it is.

We use a sample of 7 leatherbacks, whose average mass is found to be $\bar{x} = 1,045$ pounds, with a standard deviation $s = 67$ pounds. We assume that the mass X of a randomly chosen Atlantic leatherback has a normal distribution. To perform the test, we calculate the ratio:

$$t_0 = \frac{\bar{x} - \mu_0}{s/\sqrt{n}} = \frac{1,045 - 1,000}{67/\sqrt{7}} = 1.78.$$

To decide if the value 1.78 is sufficiently large for a random variable T with a $T(6)$ distribution, we consider:

$$p\text{-value} = P(T > 1.78).$$

Searching on row $\nu = 7 - 1 = 6$ of Table 17.4 for a value close to 1.78, we find that 1.78 lies between 1.440 and 1.943, whose corresponding areas to the right are 0.10, respectively 0.05.

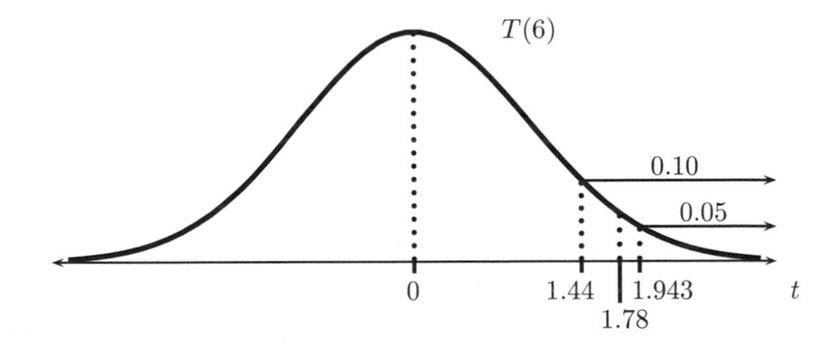

Fig. 11.2 $T(6)$ distribution

We conclude that:

$$0.05 < p\text{-value} < 0.10.$$

Using a statistical software, we see that p-value=0.063.

Suppose first that the preset value α is 0.05, i.e. we are willing to accept a risk of 5% of making a type I error. Since the p-value is higher than 0.05, we fail to reject H_0 and we conclude that there is not enough evidence that the average mass of the Atlantic leatherbacks is larger than 1,000 pounds.

Suppose next that we are willing to accept a risk of 10% of making a type I error (i.e. $\alpha = 0.10$). In this case, since the p-value is smaller than 0.10, we reject H_0 in favor of H_1, and conclude that the average mass of the Atlantic leatherbacks is larger than 1,000 pounds.

Case (2). $H_0 : \mu = \mu_0$ versus $H_1 : \mu < \mu_0$

The test is also based on the calculation of the same ratio $t_0 = (\bar{x} - \mu_0)/(s/\sqrt{n})$. A negative value of this ratio is an indication that H_1 might be true. To see if this ratio is far from 0 (compared with other values encountered from different samples), we consider the following:

$$p\text{-value} = P(T < t_0),$$

where T is a random variable with a $T(n-1)$ distribution. If the p-value is small, we reject H_0; otherwise, we fail to reject H_0.

Example 11.5. More that 20% of the world's oxygen is produced in the Amazon rainforest. The giant kapok tree (*Ceiba pentandra*) is the tallest tree in the Amazon rainforest, with a height of up to 200 feet and a trunk diameter of 9 or 10 feet. This tree is host to numerous aerial plants, insects and birds. The average growth rate of the giant kapok tree is 10 feet per year. Researchers fear that in the past years, the growth rate of this tree has slowed down, due to climate change and deforestation. We want to test this claim, assuming that the growth rate X of a randomly chosen tree has a normal distribution with unknown mean μ. A sample of 15 giant kapok trees yielded an average annual growth $\bar{x} = 8.5$ feet, and a sample standard deviation $s = 2.1$ feet. The hypotheses to be confronted are:

$$H_0 : \mu = 10 \quad \text{versus} \quad H_1 : \mu < 10.$$

Type I error occurs when we decide that the annual growth rate has decreased, when in fact it did not. Type II error occurs when we decide that the annual growth rate has stayed the same, when in fact it has decreased.

To perform the test, we first observe that $\bar{x} = 8.5 < \mu_0 = 10$. Hence, we can proceed in the direction of H_1. For this, we calculate the ratio:

$$t_0 = \frac{\bar{x} - \mu_0}{s/\sqrt{n}} = \frac{8.5 - 10}{2.1/\sqrt{15}} = -2.77.$$

In this case,

$$p\text{-value} = P(T < -2.77) = P(T > 2.77),$$

where T is a random variable with a $T(14)$ distribution. Note that for the second equality above, we used the symmetry of the $T(14)$ distribution. Looking on row $\nu = 14$ of Table 17.4, we see that 2.77 lies between the values 2.624 and 2.977, whose corresponding areas to the right are 0.01, respectively 0.005. Hence,

$$0.005 < p\text{-value} < 0.01.$$

Using a statistical software, we see that p-value=0.008.

Since the p-value is smaller than $\alpha = 0.01$, we reject H_0 and conclude that the annual growth rate of the kapok tree has slowed down.

Case (3). $H_0 : \mu = \mu_0$ versus $H_1 : \mu \neq \mu_0$

As in Case (3) of Section 11.1, we calculate the absolute value of t_0. The p-value formula uses both tails of the $T(n-1)$ distribution and the symmetry of this distribution (which explains the 2 in the formula below):

$$p\text{-value} = 2P(T > |t_0|).$$

As in the previous two cases, we have to obtain a small p-value, in order to reject H_0 in favor of H_1.

Example 11.6. Measurements of blood viscosity were made on laboratory mice. A normal value should be close to 3.95. Researchers who are testing a new drug suspect that this could have modified their blood viscosity level, but they do not know the direction of this change. Levels which are either too small or too large are not acceptable. We want to see if there is enough evidence that the average level of viscosity has deviated significantly from the value 3.95, due to the new drug. We are interested in testing:

$$H_0 : \mu = 3.95 \quad \text{versus} \quad H_1 : \mu \neq 3.95,$$

where μ is the average viscosity level for the mice which were treated with the new drug.

A type I error occurs when we decide that the viscosity level is affected by the new drug, when in fact it is not. A type II error occurs when we fail to gain evidence that the drug affects the viscosity level, when in fact it does.

A sample of 9 mice yields a sample viscosity level $\bar{x} = 5.25$ and a sample standard deviation $s = 0.6$. We calculate the ratio:

$$t_0 = \frac{\bar{x} - \mu_0}{s/\sqrt{n}} = \frac{5.25 - 3.95}{0.6/\sqrt{9}} = 6.50$$

and then,

$$p\text{-value} = 2P(T > 6.50),$$

where T is a random variable with a $T(8)$ distribution. Looking on row $\nu = 9 - 1 = 8$ of Table 17.4, we see that 6.50 is larger than the last value listed in the table, namely 3.355 (whose corresponding area to the right is 0.005). Hence, $P(T > 6.5) < 0.005$ and

$$p\text{-value} < 2(0.005) = 0.01.$$

Using a statistical software, we see that p-value=0.0002.

Since the p-value is very small, we reject H_0 and conclude that the new drug affects the blood viscosity level.

We should point out that in practice, if the sample size is large (i.e. $n \geq 40$), one may replace T by a standard normal random variable Z, in the calculation of the p-value. This is called a *large sample test* and is justified by the fact that the distribution of T_0 becomes approximately standard normal, when n is large enough (see Theorem 9.5).

11.3 Hypothesis Testing for the Proportion

In this section, we are interested in confronting two hypotheses which speak about the value of the proportion p of individuals who share a common characteristic in a given population. Recall from Section 9.2, that an estimate for p is:

$$\hat{p} = \frac{y}{n}$$

where y denotes the number of individuals with the desired characteristic, in a sample of size n.

Example 11.7. A recent article in the National Geographic magazine (April 2009) draws attention on a form of fungal infection, chytridiomycosis (chytrid for short), which is wiping out amphibians on all continents where frogs live. The Amphibian Ark is an international project aimed at keeping at least 500 amphibian species in captivity for reintroduction when the crisis is resolved. In the wild, an infection rate higher that 90% is critical for a species to survive. Researchers suspect that this rate has already been attained for the mountain yellow-legged frogs of the Sixty Lake Basin in California's Sierra Nevada. In a sample of 85 frogs, 77 tested positive for the chytrid fungus. We want to test the hypotheses:

$$H_0 : p = 0.90 \quad \text{versus} \quad H_1 : p > 0.90,$$

where p is the percentage of mountain yellow-legged frogs in the Sixty Lake Basin, which are infected by chytrid. An estimate for p is:

$$\hat{p} = \frac{77}{85} = 0.906, \quad \text{or} \quad 90.6\%.$$

A type I error occurs when we decide that the infection rate exceeds the critical rate of 90%, when in fact it does not. A type II error occurs when we fail to show that the infection rate exceeds the critical rate of 90%, when in fact it does.

Example 11.8. Topiramate (commonly known as topamax in Canada and the United States) was approved for use as a treatment for epilepsy in 1995. In 2004, the American Food and Drug Administration approved the drug for use in treating migraines. Side effects of topiramate treatment include fatigue, nausea and confusion. We want to gain evidence for the fact that these side effects appear in less than 6% of the population. In a group of 150 patients treated with topiramate, only 6 complained about side effects. We would like to test the hypotheses:

$$H_0 : p = 0.06 \quad \text{versus} \quad H_1 : p < 0.06,$$

where p is the (unknown) proportion of people who experience side effects, among those who are using topiramate. An estimate for p is:

$$\hat{p} = \frac{6}{150} = 0.04, \quad \text{or} \quad 4\%.$$

A type I error occurs when we decide that the percentage of people who experience side effects is lower than 6%, when in fact it is not. A type II error occurs when we fail to show that the percentage of people who experience side effects is lower that 6%, when in fact it is.

Example 11.9. Conventional detergents are based on petrochemicals which are rapidly depleting sources of non-renewable materials, and whose residues are poorly biodegradable, building up in the environment. By contrast, ecological detergents are biodegradable, being produced using ingredients of renewable origin. The effectiveness of ecological detergents in removing oil stains is thought to be around 80%. A new ecological detergent was used in a sample of 500 laundry loads containing oil stained items. 435

loads resulted in the complete removal of oil stains. Based on this sample, we want to test the hypothesis:

$$H_0 : p = 0.80 \quad \text{versus} \quad H_1 : p \neq 0.80,$$

where p is the effectiveness in removing oil stains of the ecological detergent. An estimate for p is:

$$\hat{p} = \frac{435}{500} = 0.87, \quad \text{or} \quad 87\%.$$

A type I error occurs when we decide that the effectiveness of the new detergent is significantly different then 80%, when in fact it is not. A type II error occurs when we fail to show that the effectiveness of the new detergent is different then 80%, when in fact it is.

We consider the following three cases:

Case (1). $H_0 : p = p_0$ versus $H_1 : p > p_0$

In this case, we want to show that the unknown proportion p is higher than a fixed numerical value p_0. To move in this direction, first we have to make sure that the estimate $\hat{p}$ is larger than p_0. A large difference between $\hat{p}$ and p_0 is a good sign in favor of H_1. The next question is: how large the difference $\hat{p} - p_0$ should be, to comfortably reject H_0? To answer this question, we use fact that, if H_0 is true then

$$Z_0 = \frac{\hat{p} - p_0}{\sqrt{p_0(1 - p_0)/n}} \quad \text{has approximately a } N(0,1) \text{ distribution,}$$

if n is large.

Our decision is based on the observed value of the test statistic:

$$z_0 = \frac{\hat{p} - p_0}{\sqrt{p_0(1 - p_0)/n}}.$$

A large value of this ratio is an indication that H_1 might be true. The idea is to compare this ratio against all other possible values (which may arise from different samples), by means of the p-value. In this case,

$$p\text{-value} = P(Z > z_0).$$

The smaller the p-value, the less likely it is that H_0 is true. We reject H_0 (and gain evidence for H_1), if the p-value is very small.

Example 11.7 (Continued). In this case, $\hat{p} = 0.906$, $n = 85$ and $p_0 = 0.90$. We calculate the observed value of the test statistic:

$$z_0 = \frac{\hat{p} - p_0}{\sqrt{p_0(1 - p_0)/n}} = \frac{0.906 - 0.90}{\sqrt{(0.90)(0.10)/85}} = 0.18.$$

The p-value is:

$$p\text{-value} = P(Z > 0.18) = 1 - 0.5714 = 0.4286.$$

Since the p-value is large, we cannot reject H_0. We conclude that there is not enough evidence that the infection rate is higher than 90%.

Case (2). $H_0 : p = p_0$ versus $H_1 : p < p_0$

To move in the direction of H_1, the estimate $\hat{p}$ has to be smaller than p_0. The testing procedure is based on the same ratio z_0 as in Case (1). In this case, the ratio is negative, and the p-value is:

$$p\text{-value} = P(Z < z_0).$$

We reject H_0 if the p-value is small.

Example 11.8 (Continued). Using $p_0 = 0.06$, $n = 150$, and $\hat{p} = 0.04$, we calculate the observed value of the test statistic:

$$z_0 = \frac{\hat{p} - p_0}{\sqrt{p_0(1-p_0)/n}} = \frac{0.04 - 0.06}{\sqrt{(0.06)(0.94)/150}} = -1.03.$$

Using Table 17.2, we obtain:

$$p\text{-value} = P(Z < -1.03) = 0.1515.$$

Since the p-value is large, we cannot reject H_0 in favor of H_1. The conclusion is that this sample does not contain enough evidence that the percentage of people suffering side effects from topamax is smaller than 0.06.

Case (3). $H_0 : p = p_0$ versus $H_1 : p \neq p_0$

In this case, we calculate the absolute value of the ratio z_0. The p-value is:

$$p\text{-value} = 2P(Z > |z_0|).$$

As in the previous two cases, we reject H_0 in favor of H_1, if the p-value is small.

Example 11.7 (Continued). In this case $p_0 = 0.80$, $\hat{p} = 0.87$ and $n = 500$. We calculate the absolute value:

$$|z_0| = \left| \frac{\hat{p} - p_0}{\sqrt{p_0(1-p_0)/n}} \right| = \left| \frac{0.87 - 0.80}{\sqrt{(0.80)(0.20)/500}} \right| = 3.91.$$

Using Table 17.3, we see that:

$$p\text{-value} = 2P(Z > 3.91) < 2(0.0001) = 0.0002.$$

(We used the fact that the value 3.91 is larger than the largest value given in Table 17.3, namely 3.89, whose area to the right is 0.0001.) Since the p-value is very small, we reject H_0 and conclude that the efficiency of the new ecological detergent is different than 0.80.

11.4 Problems

Problem 11.1. The Greenland ice sheet covers roughly 80% of the surface of Greenland, being the second largest body of ice in the world, after the Antarctic ice sheet. As the arctic climate is rapidly warming, the Greenland ice sheet has experienced record melting in the recent years. The following data gives the depth of the ice sheet (in m) measured at various locations during the summer months in the Northeast Greenland National Park:

3115 3133 3123 3145 3125 3131 3127 3120 3118 3124

Using this data, is there enough evidence that the average depth of the ice sheet is below 3140m? Assume that the depth of the ice sheet is normally distributed.

Problem 11.2. The article [7] studies the acquisition of rainfall data in Guinea Savanna part of Nigeria. One of the major data acquisition problems in Sub-Saharan Africa includes instrumental errors, which are associated with the functioning of the instruments. An error encountered frequently with the rain gauges (instruments used by hydrologists) occurs during the siphoning cycle, when the rain persists to enter the rain gauge. Assume that the measurement error is a normal random variable with unknown mean μ and known standard deviation $\sigma = 0.5$ mm. In a sample of 16 observations, it was found that the mean measurement error was $\bar{x} = 0.28$ mm. Is there enough evidence that the average measurement error μ exceeds the threshold of 0.25 mm?

Problem 11.3. Refer to Problem 10.6. Using these data, is there enough evidence to conclude that the mean yield has increased, compared to the average yield of 2.7 kg per year?

Problem 11.4. Refer to Problem 6.5. Using these data, is there enough evidence to conclude that the use of this medication is better than not using any medication for reducing pain? (Hint: Use the binomial distribution to compute the p-value, since the sample size is small.)

Problem 11.5. For many years a farmer has not kiln-dry his barley seeds before sowing. (To kiln-dry means to dry in an insulated chamber where airflow, temperature and humidity are controlled.) The non-kiln-dried seeds yield on average 672 kg of barley per 4000 m^2. This year the farmer decides to kiln-dry his barley seeds before sowing. Ten varieties of kiln-dried barley seeds are sown. The yields (in kg per 4000 m^2) are below.

652.3	706.1	679.9	630.9	664.0	647.5	697.6	686.8	722.6	655.0

(a) Using these data, is there enough evidence to conclude that the mean yield has increased? (First verify that the yields are normally distributed.)
(b) Construct a 95% confidence interval for the mean yield of kiln-dried barley.

Problem 11.6. Refer to Problem 10.8. Is there enough evidence to conclude that the new drug has a larger rate of effectiveness compared to another drug, which is effective in 66% of the cases? Use a test of hypothesis at the significance level $\alpha = 0.10$.

Did you know that? *William Gosset was a student of both chemistry and mathematics. He also worked and studied during the period of 1906-1907 in the biometrics laboratory of Karl Pearson at University College London. The Student distribution was discovered by Gosset while working as a brewer and scientist at Guinness in the early 20th century. Guinness prohibited its employees from publishing, so Gosset used the pseudonym Student. While performing quality control for Guinness, Gosset saw the need for developing statistical methods for small samples, i.e. methods that do not rely on asymptotic results such as the Central Limit Theorem. He was able to guess the form of the density of the studentization of the sample mean* $(\overline{X}-\mu)/(S/\sqrt{n})$*, under the assumption that the population is normal. He used mathematical arguments and empirical work (experiments) to construct the T-distribution. Gosset's results were confirmed later by Ronald Fisher. Fisher appreciated the importance of Gosset's small-sample work, which inspired much of his own work.*

Chapter 12

Comparison of Two Independent Samples

Biologists are often interested in the comparison of groups. Consider the following examples. Do two different species of swallow produce similar eggs on average? Does a type of fertilizer produce larger plants on average, compared to another type of fertilizer? In this chapter, we introduce methods to compare two independent groups. We discuss how interval estimation and hypothesis testing can be used to infer whether there are differences between the two populations. We first discuss techniques to compare means, and end the chapter with techniques to compare proportions.

12.1 Study/Experimental Design

When analyzing data, it is important to consider the design of the study or experiment. This is especially true when comparing groups. The design of the study often dictates the probability model that will be used to describe the data collection process from the populations of interest. It is only when the probability model is appropriate, that we can generalize our results from the samples to the populations.

Scientists often want to compare groups that are outcomes from a controlled experiment which is run under different experimental conditions. For example, a simple experiment might be designed to test a claim that a particular type of fertilizer produces taller plants compared to another type of fertilizer. The response variable in this instance is the height of the plants. The primary factor for this experiment is the fertilizer. The levels of the factor are called *treatments*. So the treatments in this case are the types of fertilizer. In a controlled experiment we assign the treatments to the experimental units, which could be plots with one seedling in this case. This assignment determines the treatment groups.

It is possible that there are uncontrolled factors that might affect the response variable. These are called *nuisance factors.* For example the genetic predisposition of a seedling to produce a tall plant might be a nuisance factor. *Randomization* is used to average the effects of the nuisance factors over the different groups. We should randomly assign the types of fertilizer to the seedlings.

The purpose of a controlled experiment is to determine if there is a *cause-and-effect* relationship. In our case, this means that the use of the new fertilizer produces taller plants on average. If the controlled experiment is randomized and the treatment groups are statistically significantly different, then we can be confident that there is indeed a cause-and-effect relationship.

One of the simplest experimental designs is called a *completely randomized design.* For completely randomized designs, the levels of the primary factor are randomly assigned to the experimental units. Our fertilizer experiment has such a design. The tools introduced in this chapter apply to experiments with a completely randomized design.

In some circumstances, the distribution of the response variable can be highly spread-out. This variability might be due to nuisance factors. For example, females and males might react differently to a particular drug. This noise can be prohibitive, in the sense that we would need very large samples in order to identify significant treatment effects. To reduce this noise we can construct homogeneous subgroups, called *blocks.* The variance within each block should be smaller than the variance of the entire sample. So the estimates within the blocks should be more precise. As we combine the estimates across blocks, we should obtain an estimate of the treatment effect that is more precise than without *blocking.*

If we randomly assign all of the treatments to the experimental units within each block, then we say that the experiment has a *randomized complete block design.* As an example, if we want to compare a drug to a placebo and we believe that the gender has also an effect on the response, we divide the subjects into blocks according to their gender. If we have ten subjects of each gender, we randomly assign the drug to five subjects of each gender. The remainder of the subjects are given the placebo. We do not discuss the analysis of block designs in this chapter.

The techniques presented in this chapter do not apply only to completely randomized experiments. They are also applicable in a non-experimental setting. Consider the study [55], where the authors compare the breeding biology of the Welcome Swallow in Australia and New Zealand. The factor (in this case, the location) is not assigned to the unit of study (the bird). Such a study is called an *observational study.*

An observational study can identify associations, but not causality. We are not randomly assigning the treatments to the units of study. So there is a danger that any association that we find between the response and the factor may be due to some third variable, called a *lurking* variable, which is not evenly distributed among the groups. Maybe it is access to food that caused the difference in breeding biology, and not the location. So we should not say that it is the observational factor that caused the significant result. However, we can say that there is an association.

The techniques in this chapter can be used to compare samples from an observational study as long as it is reasonable to assume that observations within the samples are independent, and that there is independence between the two samples.

12.2 Confidence Intervals and Tests for Means

In this section, we discuss techniques to compare the means of two independent populations. We use X_1 and X_2 to denote the random measurements from population 1 and population 2, respectively. Their means are denoted by $\mu_1 = E(X_1)$ and $\mu_2 = E(X_2)$ and their variances are denoted by $\sigma_1^2 = \text{Var}(X_1)$ and $\sigma_2^2 = \text{Var}(X_2)$. We assume that we have a random sample of size n_1 from population 1, and a random sample of size n_2 from population 2.

To compare the two means, we examine the difference in means $\mu_1 - \mu_2$. We consider four cases: (1) normal (or general) population with known variances σ_1^2 and σ_2^2 (large samples sizes are needed if the populations are not normal); (2) normal population with unknown but equal variances ($\sigma_1^2 = \sigma_2^2$), and (possibly) small sample sizes; (3) normal population with unknown and unequal variances ($\sigma_1^2 \neq \sigma_2^2$), and (possibly) small sample sizes; and (4) general populations with unknown variances and large sample sizes.

We begin the discussion with point estimation. A natural estimator of $\mu_1 - \mu_2$ is the difference in sample means $\overline{X}_1 - \overline{X}_2$. This estimator is unbiased since its expected value is $E(\overline{X}_1 - \overline{X}_2) = \mu_1 - \mu_2$. The variance of the estimator is

$$\text{Var}(\overline{X}_1 - \overline{X}_2) = \frac{\sigma_1^2}{n_1} + \frac{\sigma_2^2}{n_2}.$$

Similar to the estimation of the mean in the one sample case, the larger the sample sizes, the more precise is the estimate. Furthermore, as we standardize $\overline{X}_1 - \overline{X}_2$, we obtain that

$$\frac{\overline{X}_1 - \overline{X}_2 - (\mu_1 - \mu_2)}{\sqrt{\sigma_1^2/n_1 + \sigma_2^2/n_2}} \text{ has a } N(0,1) \text{ distribution.} \tag{12.1}$$

The test statistics that we introduce in this section are based upon (and are slight modifications) of the standardization (12.1).

We consider the inference concerning the difference $\mu_1 - \mu_2$. The null hypothesis is of the form $H_0 : \mu_1 - \mu_2 = \delta_0$, where δ_0 is a given numeric value. Note that when $\delta_0 = 0$, the null hypothesis becomes $H_0 : \mu_1 - \mu_2 = 0$, or equivalently $H_0 : \mu_1 = \mu_2$.

Case (1). Normal (or General) Populations with Known Variances σ_1^2 and σ_2^2.

This case is usually not encountered in practice. We discuss it mainly for theoretical purposes. In this case, we use the following test statistic:

$$Z_0 = \frac{\overline{X}_1 - \overline{X}_2 - \delta_0}{\sqrt{\sigma_1^2/n_1 + \sigma_2^2/n_2}}. \tag{12.2}$$

If H_0 holds, then the sampling distribution of Z_0 is a standard normal. Hence we can use Table 17.3, to compute the corresponding p-value. Recall that the p-value is the probability of observing a value as extreme as the current observed value, under the assumption that the null hypothesis holds. Since our definition of an extreme value depends on the alternative hypothesis, the computation of the p-value depends on the alternative hypothesis.

Note that, when both samples are large, the standardized difference given by (12.1) follows approximately a standard normal distribution, even if the populations are not normally distributed. (This is an application of the Central Limit Theorem; see Theorem 9.5.)

Table 12.1 gives the p-value for testing the null hypothesis $H_0 : \mu_1 - \mu_2 = \delta_0$ against one of the alternative hypotheses H_1. In this table, Z has a standard normal distribution and $z_0 = (\overline{x}_1 - \overline{x}_2 - \delta_0)/\sqrt{\sigma_1^2/n_1 + \sigma_2^2/n_2}$ is the observed value of the test statistic Z_0 given by (12.2).

The p-value is a measure of how much evidence we have against the null hypothesis. The smaller the p-value, the greater the inconsistency between the data and the null hypothesis. Actually, the p-value is the smallest level of significance at which the null hypothesis can be rejected

Table 12.1 The p-value in Case (1)

Alternative Hypothesis	p-value
$H_1 : \mu_1 - \mu_2 > \delta_0$	$P(Z > z_0)$
$H_1 : \mu_1 - \mu_2 < \delta_0$	$P(Z < z_0)$
$H_1 : \mu_1 - \mu_2 \neq \delta_0$	$2\,P(Z > \lvert z_0 \rvert)$

with the given data. If the p-value is smaller than α, then we reject the null hypothesis in favor of the alternative hypothesis. When the null hypothesis $H_0 : \mu_1 - \mu_2 = 0$ is rejected, it is often said that the difference between μ_1 and μ_2 is statistically significant.

The p-value is a valuable statistic that measures the risk associated with rejecting the null hypothesis. However, it does not give us the whole picture. Think of the hypothesis test as a diagnostic tool. We must assess its specificity and its sensitivity (often called *power* in the context of hypothesis testing). We can control its specificity (our chances of failing to reject H_0 when H_0 is true) with the use of a significance level. We can use a confidence interval to assess the sensitivity (our chances of rejecting H_0 when H_1 is true).

A confidence interval is also useful as a stand-alone tool if the goal is simply to estimate the difference in means. A confidence interval for $\mu_1 - \mu_2$ at a level of confidence of $(1 - \alpha)\,100\%$ is

$$\overline{x}_1 - \overline{x}_2 \pm z\sqrt{\frac{\sigma_1^2}{n_1} + \frac{\sigma_2^2}{n_2}}$$

where z is a value such that $P(-z < Z < z) = 1 - \alpha$ and Z follows a standard normal distribution.

Regardless of whether the difference is found to be statistically significant or not, it is important to assess the sensitivity of the hypothesis test. This will be demonstrated through the use of examples. To assess the sensitivity of the test we must first determine practical (biological or clinical) significance. As an example, consider the comparison of mean triglyceride levels for two groups. The researcher might decide that a difference in means of 5 mg/dl is not biologically important, but a difference of 20 mg/dl is important. Researchers determine practical importance using their good judgment and experience.

Suppose that we found a statistically significant difference in the mean triglyceride levels. The researcher produces a 95% confidence interval for the difference in means and he finds that the difference in means is between 2.3 mg/dl to 4.7 mg/dl. The researcher concludes that the means are statistically different, but the difference is not biologically (or clinically) important. In this instance, the test is highly sensitive since it can detect differences in means which have no practical significance.

Now suppose a scenario where the p-value is large, so we fail to reject the null hypothesis that the means are equal. The researcher produces a 95% confidence interval for the difference in means and finds that the difference in means is between -2.5 mg/dl to 24.1 mg/dl. The maximum error of the estimate is very large. Perhaps the failure to reject the null hypothesis was caused by an inadequate sample size. The test is not sensitive (also said not powerful) enough to detect a difference of biological importance.

A large p-value should not automatically be interpreted as evidence in support of the null hypothesis, and a small p-value should not automatically be interpreted as evidence in support of practical significance. All biologists should be ultimately interested in biological importance, which may be assessed using confidence intervals.

Case (2). Normal Populations with Unknown but Equal Variances ($\sigma_1^2 = \sigma_2^2$), and (Possibly) Small Sample Sizes.

In Case (1), we discussed the inference concerning $\mu_1 - \mu_2$ for independent normal populations, under the assumption that the variances are known. In Case (2), Case (3), and Case (4), we extend these techniques to the case when the variances are unknown.

In Case (2), the underlying assumptions of our model are independent normal populations with equal but unknown variances. In addition, the sample sizes could be small. We denote the common variance by σ^2. With the added assumption of homogeneity of the variance, the standardization of the estimator $\overline{X}_1 - \overline{X}_2$ becomes

$$\frac{\overline{X}_1 - \overline{X}_2 - (\mu_1 - \mu_2)}{\sigma\sqrt{1/n_1 + 1/n_2}} \text{ has a } N(0,1) \text{ distribution.}$$

Since σ^2 is unknown, we cannot base our inference on this statistic. Denoting by S_i^2 the sample variance from population i, for $i = 1, 2$, and using the fact that $E(S_i^2) = \sigma_i^2 = \sigma^2$, this means that both S_1^2 and S_2^2 are unbiased estimators of the common variance σ^2. We combine them to obtain a better estimator of σ^2. One possible combination is to take a weighted average of the variances with weights based on their respective degrees of freedom. This gives us an unbiased estimator of σ^2, known as the *pooled sample variance*:

$$S_p^2 = \frac{\nu_1}{\nu_1 + \nu_2} S_1^2 + \frac{\nu_2}{\nu_1 + \nu_2} S_2^2 = \frac{(n_1 - 1)S_1^2 + (n_2 - 1)S_2^2}{n_1 + n_2 - 2},$$

where $\nu_i = n_i - 1$, for $i = 1, 2$. The pooled sample standard deviation is $S_p = \sqrt{S_p^2}$. As we replace σ by S_p in the standardization of $\overline{X}_1 - \overline{X}_2$, we get the following studentization:

$$\frac{\overline{X}_1 - \overline{X}_2 - (\mu_1 - \mu_2)}{S_p\sqrt{1/n_1 + 1/n_2}} \text{ has a } T(n_1 + n_2 - 2) \text{ distribution.} \tag{12.3}$$

A $(1-\alpha)\,100\%$ confidence interval for $\mu_1 - \mu_2$ is

$$\overline{x}_1 - \overline{x}_2 \pm t\, s_p \sqrt{\frac{1}{n_1} + \frac{1}{n_2}},$$

where t is a value such that $P(-t < T < t) = 1 - \alpha$, and T has a $T(n_1 + n_2 - 2)$ distribution. For testing $H_0 : \mu_1 - \mu_2 = \delta_0$, we use the test statistic:

$$T_0 = \frac{\overline{X}_1 - \overline{X}_2 - \delta_0}{S_p\sqrt{1/n_1 + 1/n_2}}.$$

If H_0 is true, T_0 has a $T(n_1 + n_2 - 2)$ distribution. A hypothesis test based on this test statistic is called *Student's two-sample t-test.* The p-value is given in Table 12.2, where $t_0 = (\overline{x}_1 - \overline{x}_2)/(s_p\sqrt{1/n_1 + 1/n_2})$ is the observed value of the test statistic T_0, and T has a $T(n_1 + n_2 - 2)$ distribution.

Table 12.2 The p-value in Case (2)

Alternative Hypothesis	p-value
$H_1 : \mu_1 - \mu_2 > \delta_0$	$P(T > t_0)$
$H_1 : \mu_1 - \mu_2 < \delta_0$	$P(T < t_0)$
$H_1 : \mu_1 - \mu_2 \neq \delta_0$	$2\,P(T > \lvert t_0 \rvert)$

Example 12.1. An agriculture researcher wants to test the claim that on average, a new fertilizer yields taller plants at maturity. A completely randomized design is used to generate the data. Sixteen similar plots with one seedling (the experimental units) are randomly assigned to the treatments, which in this case are the new and the old fertilizer. A balance design is used, i.e. both treatment groups are of equal size. The plants are measured at maturity (in cm). Here are the data:

Old Fertilizer	New Fertilizer
46.1	49.8
37.7	51.5
54.2	50.7
44.7	50.7
30.9	41.9
38.5	36.4
38.0	59.4
55.0	41.9

summary data

size	mean	variance
$n_1 = 8$	$\overline{x}_1 = 43.14$	$s_1^2 = 71.65$
$n_2 = 8$	$\overline{x}_2 = 47.79$	$s_2^2 = 52.66$

The researcher wants to test $H_0 : \mu_1 - \mu_2 = 0$ against $H_1 : \mu_1 - \mu_2 < 0$ using Student's two-sample t-test.

Figure 12.1 gives an overlay of the normal probability plots for the two samples. There are no systematic tendencies away from the lines, hence we do not have strong evidence against normality. Furthermore, the slopes of the lines are similar. So it appears that the equal variance assumption holds. To further assess this underlying assumption, we can also do a comparative box plot analysis (see Figure 12.1). The first sample (old fertilizer) appears to be slightly more spread out, but this difference in variability is not striking. We do not have strong evidence against the equal variance assumption. It is reasonable to assume that the populations are normal with equal variances.

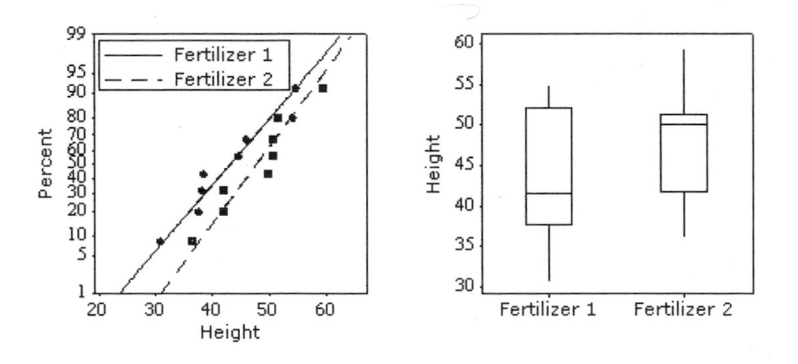

Fig. 12.1 Normal probability plots and comparative box plots for the plant heights

The pooled sample variance and standard deviation are

$$s_p^2 = \frac{(n_1 - 1)\, s_1^2 + (n_2 - 1)\, s_2^2}{n_1 + n_2 - 2} = 62.155 \quad \text{and} \quad s_p = \sqrt{62.155} = 7.8838.$$

The observed test statistic is

$$t_0 = \frac{\overline{x}_1 - \overline{x}_2}{s_p\sqrt{1/n_1 + 1/n_2}} = \frac{43.14 - 47.79}{7.8338\, \sqrt{1/8 + 1/8}} = -1.18.$$

The p-value is $P(T < t_0) = P(T < -1.18) = P(T > 1.18)$, where T has a $T(n_1 + n_2 - 2) = T(14)$ distribution. Referring to row $\nu = 14$ in Table 17.4, 1.18 falls between 0.692 and 1.345, which have areas to the right of 0.25 and 0.10. Thus, $0.10 < p$-value < 0.25. Using a statistical package, we see that p-value $= 0.129$.

At a significance level of $\alpha = 0.05$, we cannot reject H_0. The data do not appear to support the hypothesis that the use of the new fertilizer produces taller plants.

A 95% confidence interval for $\mu_1 - \mu_2$ is

$$\overline{x}_1 - \overline{x}_2 \pm t\, s_p \sqrt{\frac{1}{n_1} + \frac{1}{n_2}} = -4.65 \pm 8.4554 = [-13.11, 3.81],$$

where $t = 2.145$ satisfies $95\% = P(-t < T < t)$ and T follows a $T(14)$ distribution. We are 95% confident that the difference in means is from -13.11 cm to 3.81 cm. We are highly confident that the absolute difference in means is not larger than 14 cm. However we cannot say the same about 5 cm, since -5 lies in the confidence interval.

In the next example, we see that we can sometimes use a log-transformation to satisfy the underlying conditions to use Student's two-sample t-test.

Example 12.2. Dichloromethane is a volatile liquid that is widely used as a solvent. A chemical engineer wants to compare the dichloromethane concentration at two treatment water plants near industrial facilities. She suspects that the distributions of the dichloromethane concentration are skewed to the right due to occasional higher discharges from the industrial facilities. She verifies her hunch with histograms (see Figure 12.2).

She decides to apply a log transformation, that is, the new measurements are read in $\ln(\mu g/L)$. The normal probability plots for the data in the original scale and the log scale are given in Figure 12.3. It is evident

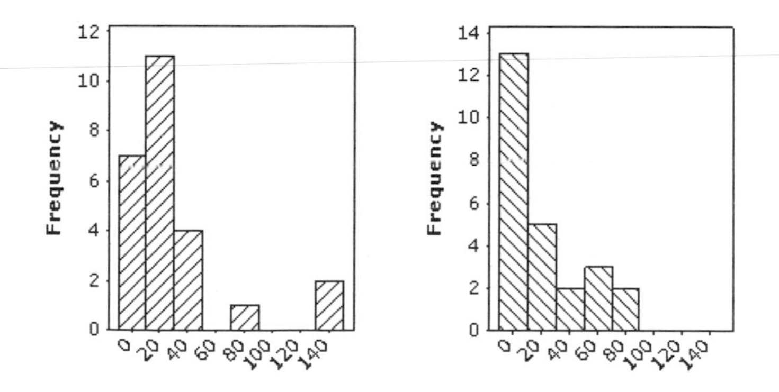

Fig. 12.2 Histograms for the dichloromethane concentrations from plants 1 and 2

from the normal probability plots that the data in the original scale are not normal, and furthermore, it appears that the variances are not equal. However, the log data appears to be normal and the variances appear to be equal since the lines in the probability plots are nearly parallel. It is safe to assume that the log concentrations from the two plants follow normal distributions with equal variances.

To compare the dichloromethane concentration at the two plants, the chemical engineer tests $H_0 : \mu_1 - \mu_2 = 0$ against $H_1 : \mu_1 - \mu_2 \neq 0$, where μ_i is the mean of the log concentrations from plant i, for $i = 1, 2$. The summary data for the log concentrations are

plant	n	$\overline{x}$	s^2
1	25	2.934	1.162
2	25	2.664	1.209

The pooled sample variance is

$$s_p^2 = \frac{(n_1 - 1)\, s_1^2 + (n_2 - 1)\, s_2^2}{n_1 + n_2 - 2} = 1.1855.$$

The observed value of Student's two sample t-test statistic is

$$t_0 = \frac{\overline{x}_1 - \overline{x}_2}{s_p \sqrt{1/n_1 + 1/n_2}} = 0.88.$$

The p-value is $2P(T > |t_0|) = 2\,P(T > 0.88)$, where T follows a $T(n_1 + n_2 - 2) = T(48)$ distribution. We cannot find the range of the p-value, using Table 17.4, since this table does not include the row $\nu = 48$. We can

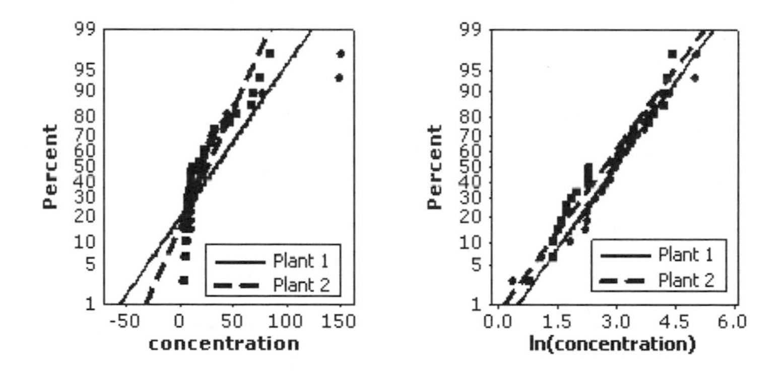

Fig. 12.3 Normal probability plots for the concentrations and log-concentrations

approximate the p-value using the row $\nu = \infty$. The approximate interval is $0.2 < p\text{-value} < 0.5$. Using a statistical software the chemical engineer computed p-value$= 0.385$. Since the p-value is large, we should not reject the hypothesis that the mean log-concentrations are the same. It appears that the means of the log concentrations are not different.

In Example 12.2, we transformed the data using a logarithm. We did this because Student's two-sample t-test requires that the populations follow a normal distribution. After inspecting the transformed data, the samples appeared to come from normal populations with equal variances, thus we could safely compare the means of the transformed data with Student's two sample t-test.

Note that, when comparing the means of the log transformed data, we are actually comparing the geometric means of the data on the original scale. To clarify the distinction between the mean and the geometric mean (for the population or the sample), we introduce the following definition.

Definition 12.1. Let $X_1, X_2, \ldots, X_n$ be a random sample from a population represented by the random variable X. The **geometric mean** of the population is $G = e^{\mu}$, where $\mu = E(\ln X)$. An estimate for G is the **(sample) geometric mean** defined by $g = e^{(1/n)\sum_{i=1}^{n} \ln x_i}$, where $x_1, \ldots, x_n$ are the observed values of the random sample $X_1, \ldots, X_n$.

Example 12.2 (Continued). We construct a 95% confidence interval for the difference in means of the log-concentrations for the data from Example 12.2. Since it is reasonable to assume that the two populations of log-concentrations are independent and normally distributed with equal variances, then a 95% confidence interval for $\mu_1 - \mu_2$ is

$$\overline{x}_1 - \overline{x}_2 \pm t\, s_p \sqrt{\frac{1}{n_1} + \frac{1}{n_2}} = 0.270 \pm 0.61930 = [-0.349, 0.889],$$

where $t = 2.011$ satisfies $95\% = P(-t < T < t)$ and T follows a $T(48)$ distribution. (The value of $t = 2.011$ was obtained using a statistical package.) We are 95% confident that $\mu_1 - \mu_2$ is between -0.349 and 0.889 (in $\ln(\mu g/L)$). Since 0 lies within the confidence interval, the means of the log-concentrations do not appear to be different.

We denote by G_i the geometric mean of the population i, consisting of the dichloromethane concentrations (in $\mu g/L$) from plant i, for $i = 1, 2$. Note that $G_i = e^{\mu_i}$, where μ_i is the mean of the log-concentration from plant i, for $i = 1, 2$. Exponentiating the difference in means gives us the ratio of the geometric means, that is $e^{\mu_1-\mu_2} = e^{\mu_1}/e^{\mu_2} = G_1/G_2$. Since we are 95% confident that $-0.349 < \mu_1 - \mu_2 < 0.889$, then we are also 95% confident that $0.71 = e^{-0.349} < G_1/G_2 < e^{0.889} = 2.43$. Since 1 lies within the interval, there appears to be no difference between the geometric means of the concentrations.

Case (3). Independent Normal Populations with Unknown and Unequal Variances ($\sigma_1^2 \neq \sigma_2^2$), and (Possibly) Small Sample Sizes.

In Case (2), we extended the inference concerning $\mu_1 - \mu_2$ for two independent normal populations with unknown variances. To do so, we assumed that the population variances are equal. The assumption of homogeneity of variance is sometimes not reasonable. So we should try to adapt our techniques to the case of unequal variance. This is known as Behrens-Fisher problem. There are exact solutions to Behrens-Fisher problem (see [19]). These solutions are beyond the scope of this book. We present an approximate solution.

In 1938, Welch [61] proposed an approximate solution to the Behrens-Fisher problem. Welch argued that the inference concerning $\mu_1 - \mu_2$ for two independent normal population can be based on

$$\frac{\overline{X}_1 - \overline{X}_2 - (\mu_1 - \mu_2)}{\sqrt{S_1^2/n_1 + S_2^2/n_2}}, \tag{12.4}$$

which follows approximately a T distribution with ν degrees of freedom, where

$$\nu = \frac{\left(s_1^2/n_1 + s_2^2/n_2\right)^2}{\left(s_1^2/n_1\right)^2/(n_1-1) + \left(s_2^2/n_2\right)^2/(n_2-1)}. \tag{12.5}$$

Since the number of degrees of freedom must be an integer, we round down ν to the nearest integer.

It follows that we can construct the following approximate $(1-\alpha)\,100\%$ confidence interval for $\mu_1 - \mu_2$:

$$\overline{x}_1 - \overline{x}_2 \pm t\sqrt{\frac{s_1^2}{n_1} + \frac{s_2^2}{n_2}},$$

where $P(-t \leq T \leq t) = 1 - \alpha$ and T has a $T(\nu)$ distribution.

To test $H_0 : \mu_1 - \mu_2 = \delta_0$, we use the test statistic

$$T_0 = \frac{\overline{X}_1 - \overline{X}_2 - \delta_0}{\sqrt{S_1^2/n_1 + S_2^2/n_2}}.$$

A test based on this test statistic is often called *Welch's approximate two-sample t-test.* This test is sometimes also called the Welch–Satterthwaite t-test or the Satterthwaite t-test. The p-value of this test is given in Table 12.3, where t_0 is the observed value of T_0, T has a $T(\nu)$ distribution, and ν is given in (12.5).

Table 12.3 The p-value in Case (3)

Alternative Hypothesis	p-value
$H_1 : \mu_1 - \mu_2 > \delta_0$	$P(T > t_0)$
$H_1 : \mu_1 - \mu_2 < \delta_0$	$P(T < t_0)$
$H_1 : \mu_1 - \mu_2 \neq \delta_0$	$2\,P(T > \|t_0\|)$

Welch's method is not exact, but is generally a good approximation. However, if the population variances are equal, or if the sample sizes are rather small and the population variances can be assumed to be approximately equal, it is more accurate to use Student's two-sample t-test. Furthermore, when the population variances are equal, Student's two-sample t-test is more powerful.

Example 12.3. An ornithologist wants to compare the breeding biology of two different species of swallows. In particular, she wants to compare the average egg mass (in grams). Here are the summary data:

	Sample Size	Mean	Var.
Species 1	18	1.872	0.264
Species 2	12	2.783	2.060

	Min.	Q1	Median	Q3	Max.
Species 1	0.900	1.400	1.900	2.300	2.800
Species 2	0.400	1.250	3.300	3.800	4.700

She wants to test $H_0 : \mu_1 - \mu_2 = 0$ against $H_1 : \mu_1 - \mu_2 \neq 0$, where μ_i is the mean egg mass (in grams) for species i, for $i = 1, 2$, with a two-sample t test. To verify the underlying assumptions of the test, she produced normal probability plots and comparative box plots (see Figure 12.4).

There are no systematic tendencies away from the normal probability plot lines, hence we do not have strong evidence against normality. However, the slopes of the lines are different. So it appears that the equal variance assumption may not hold. To further assess the underlying assumptions, we look at the comparative box plots. The egg mass for the second species are more spread out. It might not be sensible to assume that the population variances are equal.

She decides to use Welch's approximate two-sample t-test. The observed value of the test statistic is

$$t_0 = \frac{\overline{x}_1 - \overline{x}_2}{\sqrt{s_1^2/n_1 + s_2^2/n_2}} = -2.11.$$

The p-value is $2\,P(T > |t_0|) = 2\,P(T > 2.11)$, where T has an approximate $T(\nu)$ distribution with the following number of degrees of freedom:

$$\nu = \frac{\left(s_1^2/n_1 + s_2^2/n_2\right)^2}{\left(s_1^2/n_1\right)^2/(n_1 - 1) + \left(s_2^2/n_2\right)^2/(n_2 - 1)} = 12.89.$$

We round down the number of degrees of freedom to the nearest integer, that is $\nu = 12$. Referring to row $\nu = 12$ in Table 17.4, 2.11 falls between 1.782 and 2.179, which have areas to the right of 0.05 and 0.025, respectively. Thus, $0.05 < p\text{-value} < 0.10$. The p-value computed with a statistical package is 0.056. At a level of significance of $\alpha = 0.10$, we can accept the alternative hypothesis that the egg mass of the two species are different on average.

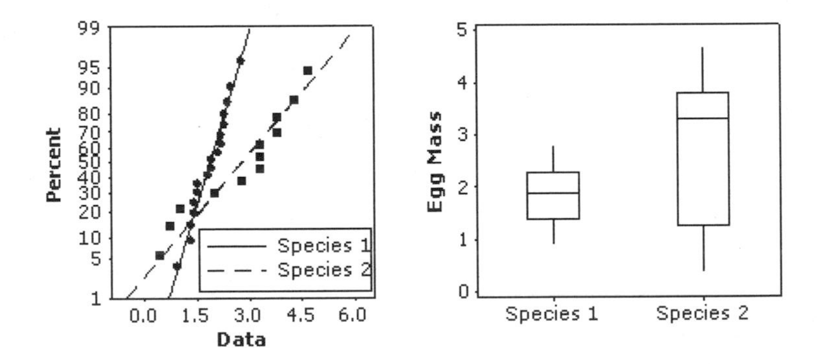

Fig. 12.4 Normal probability plots and comparative box plots for the egg masses

Case (4). General Populations with Unknown Variances, and Large Sample Sizes.

When both sample sizes are large, we can use the sample variances instead of the population variances. More precisely, to test $H_0 : \mu_1 - \mu_2 =$

δ_0, we use the test statistic

$$Z_0 = \frac{\overline{X}_1 - \overline{X}_2 - \delta_0}{\sqrt{S_1^2/n_1 + S_2^2/n_2}}.$$

Note that this is the same statistic as in Case (3), except that now we assume that its distribution is approximately normal, and therefore we use Table 17.2 or Table 17.3 for calculating the p-value (see Table 12.4). In this table, z_0 is the observed value of Z_0. This will produce a *large sample test* for comparing the means. An (approximate) $(1-\alpha)\,100\%$ confidence interval for $\mu_1 - \mu_2$ is

$$\overline{x}_1 - \overline{x}_2 \pm z\sqrt{\frac{s_1^2}{n_1} + \frac{s_2^2}{n_2}},$$

where $P(-z \leq Z \leq z) = 1 - \alpha$. We suggest not to use a large sample test or an approximate confidence interval unless both samples are at least of size 40.

Table 12.4 The p-value for Case (4)

Alternative Hypothesis	p-value
$H_1 : \mu_1 - \mu_2 > \delta_0$	$P(Z > z_0)$
$H_1 : \mu_1 - \mu_2 < \delta_0$	$P(Z < z_0)$
$H_1 : \mu_1 - \mu_2 \neq \delta_0$	$2\,P(Z > \lvert z_0 \rvert)$

Example 12.4. We want to compare the lipid content (% of weight) of the lake whitefish *Coregonus clupeaformis* in two large neighbouring lakes. The focus of the study was on medium sized fish, from 600 grams to 1,000 grams. We collected $n_1 = 175$ fish from lake 1 and $n_2 = 225$ fish from lake 2. The observed samples means and standard deviations are $\overline{x}_1 = 7.18$, $\overline{x}_2 = 7.31$, $s_1 = 0.55$ and $s_2 = 0.70$.

We test $H_0 : \mu_1 - \mu_2 = 0$ against $H_1 : \mu_1 - \mu_2 \neq 0$. The observed value of the test statistic for this large sample test is

$$z_0 = \frac{\overline{x}_1 - \overline{x}_2}{\sqrt{s_1^2/n_1 + s_2^2/n_2}} = \frac{7.18 - 7.31}{\sqrt{(0.55)^2/175 + (0.70)^2/225}} = -2.08.$$

The p-value is (approximately) equal to $2\,P(Z > |z_0|) = 2\,P(Z > 2.08) = 2\,(1 - 0.9812) = 0.0376$. At a level of significance of $\alpha = 0.05$, we can reject the hypothesis that the lake whitefish have equal mean lipid content in both lakes.

Using their good judgment and experience the researchers had determined before hand that the absolute difference $|\mu_1 - \mu_2|$ would have to be at least 1 to be of biological importance. The biological significance cannot be determined from the p-value. We must analyze the error of the estimate of $\mu_1 - \mu_2$.

A point estimate for $\mu_1 - \mu_2$ is $\overline{x}_1 - \overline{x}_2 = -0.13$ and its estimated standard error is $\sqrt{s_1^2/n_1 + s_2^2/n_2} = 0.0625$. A 95% (approximate) confidence interval for $\mu_1 - \mu_2$ is

$$\overline{x}_1 - \overline{x}_2 \pm 1.96\sqrt{\frac{s_1^2}{n_1} + \frac{s_2^2}{n_2}} = -0.13 \pm 0.1225 = [-0.25; -0.01].$$

We are 95% confident that $|\mu_1 - \mu_2| < 1$. The statistically significant difference between the means has no biological importance.

12.3 Confidence Intervals and Tests for Proportions

To compare two proportions p_1 and p_2 from two independent populations, we discuss inferences concerning the difference $p_1 - p_2$. We begin discussing the point estimation of the difference in proportions. We follow the discussion with interval estimation and hypothesis testing.

Consider two independent binomial experiments. The probability of success for the ith experiment is p_i and the number of successes is a random measurement denoted by Y_i, for $i = 1, 2$. The number of observations per experiment are n_1 and n_2, respectively. The respective sample proportions are $\widehat{p}_1 = Y_1/n_1$ and $\widehat{p}_2 = Y_2/n_2$. A natural estimator for $p_1 - p_2$ is $\widehat{p}_1 - \widehat{p}_2$. The estimator is unbiased since the expected value of the estimator is $E(\widehat{p}_1 - \widehat{p}_2) = p_1 - p_2$. The variance of this estimator is equal to

$$\mathrm{Var}(\widehat{p}_1 - \widehat{p}_2) = \mathrm{Var}(\widehat{p}_1) + \mathrm{Var}(\widehat{p}_2) = \frac{p_1(1-p_1)}{n_1} + \frac{p_2(1-p_2)}{n_2}.$$

Similar to the estimation of the difference in means, the larger the samples, the more precise the estimate. Assuming that both samples are large, as we standardize $\widehat{p}_1 - \widehat{p}_2$, we obtain that (approximately)

$$\frac{\widehat{p}_1 - \widehat{p}_2 - (p_1 - p_2)}{\sqrt{p_1(1-p_1)/n_1 + p_2(1-p_2)/n_2}} \text{ has a } N(0,1) \text{ distribution.} \qquad (12.6)$$

As in the one sample case, the latter standardization cannot be used directly since the variance is unknown (it involves the true proportions p_1 and p_2). However if we use the estimated variance, it can be shown that (approximately)

$$\frac{\widehat{p}_1 - \widehat{p}_2 - (p_1 - p_2)}{\sqrt{\widehat{p}_1(1-\widehat{p}_1)/n_1 + \widehat{p}_2(1-\widehat{p}_2)/n_2}} \text{ has a } N(0,1) \text{ distribution,} \qquad (12.7)$$

when n_1 and n_2 are large. What are large sample sizes? This is not an easy question to answer. A common rule of thumb is to not use the latter normal approximation when the observed number of successes or the observed number of failures in either one of the groups is less than 5.

Using (12.7), we construct an approximate confidence interval for $p_1 - p_2$ at a level of confidence of $(1-\alpha)\,100\%$. This interval is:

$$\widehat{p}_1 - \widehat{p}_2 \pm z\sqrt{\frac{\widehat{p}_1(1-\widehat{p}_1)}{n_1} + \frac{\widehat{p}_2(1-\widehat{p}_2)}{n_2}},$$

where z is value such that $P(-z < Z < z) = 1-\alpha$, and Z follows a standard normal distribution.

In practice, we usually want to compare our data against a model with equal proportions. In other words, we would like to test the null hypothesis $H_0 : p_1 - p_2 = 0$ (or equivalently $H_0 : p_1 = p_2$) against an appropriate alternative hypothesis. Assuming that H_0 holds, then the probability of success is the same for all trials in both experiments. This common probability is $p = p_1 = p_2$. If this is the case, we can consider the $n = n_1 + n_2$ observations as a sample from a binomial distribution with n trials and probability p of success. The corresponding sample proportion (called the *pooled sample proportion*) is

$$\widehat{p} = \frac{Y_1 + Y_2}{n} = \frac{n_1}{n}\,\widehat{p}_1 + \frac{n_2}{n}\,\widehat{p}_2.$$

Note that the pooled sample proportion is a weighted average of the respective sample proportions, where the weights are the relative sample sizes.

Assuming that H_0 is true (i.e. $p_1 = p_2$) the standardization in (12.6) becomes

$$\frac{\widehat{p}_1 - \widehat{p}_2 - 0}{\sqrt{p\,(1-p)}\,\sqrt{1/n_1 + 1/n_2}}.$$

Using $\widehat{p}$ instead of p, we get the following test statistic:

$$Z_0 = \frac{\widehat{p}_1 - \widehat{p}_2}{\sqrt{\widehat{p}\,(1-\widehat{p})}\,\sqrt{1/n_1 + 1/n_2}}.$$

Since the p-value is the probability of observing a value as extreme as z_0 (which is the observed value of the test statistic) in the direction of the alternative hypothesis, this hypothesis must be taken in consideration when computing the p-value. We usually want to test the null hypothesis of equality against one of the following three alternative forms. Table 12.5 gives the corresponding p-value in the three cases. Here Z has approximately a standard normal distribution. The test is a large sample test.

Table 12.5 The p-value for the comparison of two proportions

Alternative Hypothesis	p-value
$H_1 : p_1 - p_2 > 0$	$P(Z > z_0)$
$H_1 : p_1 - p_2 < 0$	$P(Z < z_0)$
$H_1 : p_1 - p_2 \neq 0$	$2\,P(Z > \lvert z_0 \rvert)$

Example 12.5. Refer to Example 4.7. We denote by p_1 and p_2 the proportions of recaptured moths in the light-coloured population, respectively the dark-coloured population. Among the $n_1 = 137$ light-coloured moths, $y_1 = 18$ were recaptured, whereas among the $n_2 = 493$ dark-coloured moths, $y_2 = 131$ were recaptured. The proportions of recaptured moths are: $\widehat{p}_1 = 0.131$ for the light-coloured moths, and $\widehat{p}_2 = 0.266$ for the dark-coloured moths. Is there a statistical difference between the proportions of recaptured moths, at a level of significance of $\alpha = 0.05$? If so, we wish to investigate the biological (practical) significance.

We assume that the samples are independent. Since both sample sizes are large and the observed number of successes and of failures are not too small, we can safely perform a large sample test. To test $H_0 : p_1 - p_2 = 0$ against $H_1 : p_1 - p_2 \neq 0$, we compute the test statistic:

$$\begin{aligned} z_0 &= \frac{\widehat{p}_1 - \widehat{p}_2}{\sqrt{\widehat{p}\,(1-\widehat{p})}\,\sqrt{1/n_1 + 1/n_2}} \\ &= \frac{0.131 - 0.266}{\sqrt{(0.2365)(1-0.2365)}\,\sqrt{1/137 + 1/493}} = -3.29, \end{aligned}$$

where the pooled sample proportion is

$$\widehat{p} = \frac{y_1 + y_2}{n_1 + n_2} = \frac{18 + 131}{137 + 493} = 0.2365.$$

The p-value is the probability of observing a difference in proportions as extreme as $\widehat{p}_1 - \widehat{p}_2 = -0.135$, under the assumption that both proportions are equal. This is approximately equal to $2\,P(Z > |z_0|) = 2\,P(Z > 3.29)$, where Z follows a standard normal approximately. Using Table 17.3, we can argue that that the p-value is 0.001. There is a statistical significant difference between the proportions.

To investigate the biological significance, we construct a 95% confidence interval for $p_1 - p_2$: $\widehat{p}_1 - \widehat{p}_2 \pm 1.96\,\sqrt{\widehat{p}_1(1-\widehat{p}_1)/n_1 + \widehat{p}_2(1-\widehat{p}_2)/n_2} = -0.135 \pm 0.0687 = [-0.204, -0.066]$. We are 95% confident that the difference in proportion $p_2 - p_1$ is between 6.6% to 20.4%. Recall that biological significance cannot be determined by a test. Only by using their good judgement and experience can scientists determine what is biologically significant. In this instance, if we assume that an absolute difference in proportions of at least 5% is biologically significant, then our findings are significant.

Kettlewell hypothesized that a larger proportion of the dark-coloured moths will be recaptured. We compute the corresponding p-value to test his claim. We want to test $H_0 : p_1 - p_2 = 0$ against $H_1 : p_1 - p_2 < 0$. The observed value of the test statistic is $z_0 = -3.29$. The p-value for this left-tailed test is approximately equal to $P(Z < z_0) = P(Z < -3.29)$, where Z has a standard normal distribution. Using Table 17.2, we can argue that the p-value is 0.0005.

12.4 Problems

Problem 12.1. It is believed that nutritional deprivation affects various components of the immune system, such as the tuberculin skin reactivity. In the study [50], a sample of 8 Sprague-Dawley male rats were fed with a normal diet consisting of 18% protein. A state of malnutrition was induced in another sample of 8 rats, which were fed with a diet consisting of only 5% protein. After 4 weeks, the rats were given an intradermal injection of 25 μg of purified protein derivative of tuberculin. The following table gives the skin reactivity diameter of erythema and induration (in mm) for the two groups of rats.

18% protein diet	5% protein diet
13.3	5.1
16.3	8.7
9.9	8.7
9.3	8.5
16.1	8.1
9.7	6.9
9.7	6.9
14.1	12.3

(a) Using a statistical software, verify the assumption that the two populations are normal with equal variances.
(b) Test the hypothesis $H_0 : \mu_1 = \mu_2$ versus $H_1 : \mu_1 > \mu_2$, where μ_1 is the average level of tuberculin reactivity in the rats with a normal diet, and μ_2 is the average level of tuberculin reactivity in the malnourished rats.

State your conclusion.
(c) Construct a 95% confidence interval for $\mu_1 - \mu_2$. Can we say that the skin reactivity diameter in the malnourished rats is at least 7mm smaller than in the control group?

Problem 12.2. It is claimed that the supplementation with Coenzyme Q10 (CoQ10) during pregnancy reduces the rate of pre-eclampsia, or pregnancy induced hypertension (see [56]). 235 pregnant women at risk of pre-eclampsia were randomly divided into two groups. The first group of 118 women received 200 mg of CoQ10 daily from the 20th week of pregnancy until delivery. The other group of 117 women received a placebo. 17 women in the CoQ10 group developed pre-eclampsia, compared with 30 women in the placebo group. Can we conclude that supplementation with CoQ10 reduces the risk of developing pre-eclampsia? Justify your conclusion using a test of hypothesis at significance level $\alpha = 0.05$, and a 95% confidence interval.

Problem 12.3. Rhodamine 6G (R6G) is a fluorochrome mitochondrial dye with potential use for cancer treatment. One of the objectives of the study [21] was to show that the administration of R6G during a period of hypoglycemia reduces the growth rate of the Walker 256 tumor. A group of $n_1 = 7$ rats underwent implantation of 100 mg of viable fragments of Walker 256 carcinosarcoma, and after 48 hours they were administered R6G. The animals were fasted for 24 hours prior to the drug administration and 8 hours after. After a week, the tumors were weighed yielding a sample average and a sample standard deviation $\bar{x}_1 = 3.6g$ and $s_1 = 0.3$g. A control group of $n_2 = 7$ rats which received the same tumor transplant had the sample average and sample standard deviation $\bar{x}_2 = 7.1g$ and $s_2 = 0.7$g. Can we conclude that the administration of R6G reduces the tumor growth rate? Justify your answer using a test of hypothesis and a 95% confidence interval. Assume that the two populations have normal distributions with equal variances.

Problem 12.4. Recent studies have shown that exercise is one of the most efficient ways of increasing the release of the growth hormone in children and teenagers. However, when exercise is combined with L-arginine supplementation, children seem to grow less. The height increase (in cm) in one year was recorded for two samples of 14-year old boys. The boys in the first group participated in a physical activity for at least 3 hours a week. The boys in the second group participated in the same activities, and had a supplementation of L-arginine included in their diet. The following table gives the summary of the data:

Group	size	mean	standard deviation
Exercise	$n_1 = 50$	$\bar{x}_1 = 23.5$	$s_1 = 5.6$
Exercise and L-arginine	$n_2 = 60$	$\bar{x}_2 = 21.4$	$s_2 = 6.9$

Use a large sample test to check if there is enough evidence that the L-arginine supplementation slows down the release of the growth hormone, when compared to exercise alone. Use the level $\alpha = 0.05$.

Problem 12.5. A pH level of the soil between 5.3 and 6.5 is optimal for strawberries. To measure the pH level, a field is divided into two lots. In each lot, we randomly select 20 samples of soil. The data are below.

lot 1						
5.66	5.73	5.68	5.77	5.73	5.71	5.68
5.58	6.11	5.37	5.67	5.53	5.59	5.94
5.84	5.53	5.64	5.73	5.30	5.65	

lot 2						
5.25	6.73	6.25	5.21	5.63	6.41	5.89
6.76	5.13	5.64	5.94	6.16	5.64	6.54
5.79	5.91	6.17	6.90	5.76	6.07	

(a) Using a statistical software, verify the assumption that the two populations are normally distributed.
(b) Using a statistical software, assess the assumption that the two populations have equal variances.
(c) Test the hypothesis $H_0 : \mu_1 = \mu_2$ versus $H_1 : \mu_1 \neq \mu_2$, where μ_1 is the mean pH level of the soil in lot 1, and μ_2 is the mean pH level of the soil in lot 2. State your conclusion. Use the level $\alpha = 0.05$.

Problem 12.6. The table below gives the size of human groups involved in bear-human interactions at a particular park. The interactions were classified according to the behaviour of the bear.

	behaviour	
	Inquisitive	Avoidance
mean	$\bar{x}_1 = 3.5$	$\bar{x}_2 = 2.4$
standard deviation	$s_1 = 5.2$	$s_2 = 2.3$
sample size	$n_1 = 65$	$n_2 = 55$

Can we conclude that the mean size of the human groups involved in bear interactions are different according to the behaviour of the bear? Use the level $\alpha = 0.05$. Which test did you use to compare the two means?

Problem 12.7. In a particular park it is believed that the type of behaviour observed during human-bear interactions depends on the type of location. In the front country, among 109 human-bear interactions, 35 involved a neutral or an avoidance behaviour. In the back country, among 83 human-bear interactions, 69 involved a neutral or an avoidance behaviour. Can we conclude that the proportion of human-bear interactions that are classified as a neutral or an avoidance behaviour is larger in the back country compared to the front country? Use the level $\alpha = 0.05$.

Problem 12.8. The Nobel Prize in Chemistry in 1937 was divided between Norman Haworth for his work on carbohydrates and vitamin C, and Paul Karrer for his work on carotenoids, flavins and vitamins A and B2. Vitamin C is an ascorbic acid with antioxidant properties. A study is undertaken to compare the amount of ascorbic acid (in mg) in two popular brands of vitamin C (labeled as 100 mg). The summary of the data follows:

	Brand 1	Brand 2
mean	$\overline{x}_1 = 118$	$\overline{x}_2 = 122$
standard deviation	$s_1 = 1.2$	$s_2 = 1.75$
number of tablets	$n_1 = 15$	$n_2 = 15$

Assume that the amount of ascorbic acid in a tablet is normally distributed, and the variance of this amount is the same for the two brands.
(a) Compute the pooled standard deviation for the two samples.
(b) Compute the p-value of Student's two-sample t-test to compare the mean amount of ascorbic acid per tablet for the two brands. What can we conclude?
(c) Construct a 95% confidence interval for $\mu_1 - \mu_2$, where μ_1 is the mean amount of ascorbic acid per tablet for brand 1, and μ_2 is the mean amount of ascorbic acid per tablet for brand 2.

Problem 12.9. We want to compare the germination rate of a new strain of a plant against an old strain of the same plant. Below are the data.

	Germinated	Did not germinate	Total
Old strain	125	15	140
New stain	152	8	160

(a) Can we conclude that the germination rates differ? Use the level $\alpha = 0.05$.
(b) Construct a 98% confidence interval for the difference between the germination rates.

Did you know that? *In 1923, the Nobel Prize committee credited the practical extraction of insulin to a team at the University of Toronto, and awarded the Nobel Prize in Physiology/Medicine to Frederick Banting and John James Richard Macleod for the discovery of insulin. Banting, shared his prize with his assistant Charles Best, who was chosen on a flip of coin to help him carry out the lab work in the summer of 1921. MacLeod shared the prize with the biochemist James Collip, who helped to purify the extracts from ox pancreas. The first injection of insulin was given at the Toronto General Hospital to a 14-year old dying diabetic patient in January 1922. The patent for insulin was sold to the University of Toronto for one dollar.*

Chapter 13

Paired Samples

In this chapter, we compare the means of two dependent populations using confidence intervals and hypothesis testing. Typical examples of dependent data sets are measurements made on the same individuals "before" and "after" a certain treatment: the weight before and after a diet program, the blood pressure before and after a physical exercise, etc. Other examples of dependent data sets are measurements made on the same individuals using two different treatments. In both cases, the observations come in pairs, and together they constitute a "paired sample".

13.1 Confidence Intervals for μ_D

Let $(X_1, Y_1), (X_2, Y_2), \ldots, (X_n, Y_n)$ be the paired observations made on n individuals before and after a certain treatment (or when using two different treatments). We assume that $X_1, X_2, \ldots, X_n$ is a random sample from a population whose mean is denoted by μ_X, and $Y_1, Y_2, \ldots, Y_n$ is a random sample from a population whose mean is denoted by μ_Y. We would like to compare μ_X and μ_Y by calculating a confidence interval for the difference

$$\mu_D = \mu_X - \mu_Y.$$

If this interval contains mostly positive values, then we can say that μ_X is larger than μ_Y, with a certain confidence. On the other hand, if the interval contains mostly negative values, then μ_X is smaller than μ_Y, with a certain confidence. If the interval contains both positive and negative values, no conclusion can be drawn.

We first calculate the differences $D_1 = X_1 - Y_1, D_2 = X_2 - Y_2, \ldots, D_n = X_n - Y_n$. These differences constitute a random sample from a population whose mean is μ_D. This random sample is used for drawing statistical conclusions about μ_D. We denote by $\bar{D}$ the sample average and by S_D^2 the sample variance of the difference data set, i.e.

$$\bar{D} = \frac{1}{n}\sum_{i=1}^{n} D_i \quad \text{and} \quad S_d^2 = \frac{1}{n-1}\sum_{i=1}^{n}(D_i - \bar{D})^2.$$

We denote by $\bar{d}$ and s_d^2 the observed values of $\bar{D}$ and S_d^2.

Assuming that the differences $D_1, D_2, \ldots, D_n$ are normally distributed, the $100(1-\alpha)\%$-confidence interval for μ_D is given by formula (10.7):

$$\bar{d} \pm t\left(\frac{s_d}{\sqrt{n}}\right)$$

where t is the value found in Table 17.4 such that $P(-t \leq T \leq t) = 1 - \alpha$ and T is a random variable with a $T(n-1)$ distribution.

Example 13.1. One of the standard ways of measuring the lung function is FEV_1, the forced expiratory volume in one second (the total volume of air blown in one second). The FEV_1 is different in males and females and slows down with age, with a peak of 4.5 l at the age of 25. Smoking speeds up this decline. The effects of smoking on the decline of FEV_1 are studied in [43]. In this example, we want to show that smoking cessation improves the lung function in 3 months time. The following table gives the FEV_1 values for 9 males in their mid 30's before quitting smoking (the x measurement), and 3 months after quitting (the y measurement), as well as the differences $d = x - y$:

x_i (FEV_1 before)	y_i (FEV_1 after)	Difference $d_i = x_i - y_i$
2.94	4.22	−1.28
2.90	4.12	−1.22
3.11	4.35	−1.24
2.85	4.09	−1.24
2.93	4.15	−1.22
3.00	4.29	−1.29
2.93	4.18	−1.25
3.03	4.29	−1.26
3.13	4.33	−1.2

After quitting smoking, we notice an increase in the FEV_1 measurements for all subjects. Recall from Section 9.3, that a commonly used tool for assessing the normality of a data set is the QQ-plot. Figure 13.1 gives the QQ-plot of the difference data set. Since the plot shows a linear tendency, we may assume that the difference data set has a normal distribution.

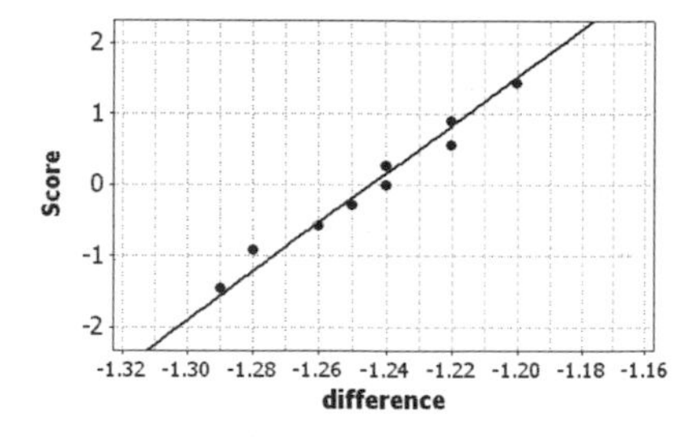

Fig. 13.1 QQ-plot of the differences between the FEV_1 levels

The sample mean and the sample standard deviation for the before/after measurements and the differences are given below:

	Before	After	Difference
Mean	$\bar{x} = 2.980$	$\bar{y} = 4.224$	$\bar{d} = -1.244$
Standard deviation	$s_x = 0.0950$	$s_y = 0.0949$	$s_d = 0.029$

Note that $\bar{x} - \bar{y} = \bar{d}$, but $s_x^2 + s_y^2 \neq s_d^2$.

To find a 95% confidence interval for the average difference between the FEV_1 after quitting smoking and before quitting smoking, we use the value $t = 2.306$, which corresponds to a T random variable with a $T(8)$ distribution, such that $P(T > 2.306) = 0.025$. This interval is:

$$-1.244 \pm 2.306 \left(\frac{0.029}{\sqrt{9}} \right) = -1.244 \pm 0.022 = [-1.266; -1.222].$$

Since the interval contains only negative values, we are 95% confident that the average difference μ_D is negative, that is the average FEV_1 value (μ_X) before quitting smoking is smaller than the average FEV_1 value (μ_Y) after quitting smoking. Based on this data, we can say that smoking cessation induces an increase of the FEV_1 value.

Example 13.2. A sample of 15 people participate in a study which compares the effectiveness of two drugs for reducing the level of the LDL (low density lipoprotein) blood cholesterol. After using the first drug for two weeks, the decrease in their cholesterol level is recorded as the x-measurement. After a pause of two months, the same individuals are administered another drug for two weeks, and the new decrease in their cholesterol level is recorded as the y-measurement. The following table gives the (x, y)-measurement pairs, together with the corresponding difference $d = x - y$. The measurements are in mg/dl.

First Drug (x_i)	Second Drug (y_i)	Difference $d_i = x_i - y_i$
13.1	12.0	1.1
12.3	7.3	5.0
10.0	11.7	−1.7
17.7	12.5	5.2
19.4	18.6	0.8
10.1	12.3	−2.2
11.5	15.2	−3.7
12.6	16.3	−3.7
9.5	10.7	−1.2
12.1	9.8	2.3
18.0	15.3	2.7
7.5	6.4	1.1
6.9	8.5	−1.6
14.5	16.4	−1.9
8.6	7.8	0.8

It appears that the differences verify the assumption of normality. The sample means and the sample standard deviations for the (x, y) measurements and the differences are given below:

	First Drug	Second Drug	Difference
Mean	$\bar{x} = 12.253$	$\bar{y} = 12.053$	$\bar{d} = 0.2$
Standard deviation	$s_x = 3.8$	$s_y = 3.711$	$s_d = 2.809$

A 90% confidence interval for μ_D is

$$0.2 \pm 1.761 \left(\frac{2.809}{\sqrt{15}} \right) = 0.2 \pm 1.277 = [-1.077;\ 1.477].$$

Here, the value $t = 1.761$ is chosen such that $P(T > t) = 0.95$, where T is a random variable with a $T(14)$-distribution. Since the interval contains both positive and negative values, we cannot conclude that the average decrease in the LDL cholesterol level caused by the first drug is larger (or smaller) than that caused by the second drug.

13.2 Hypothesis Testing for μ_D

As in the previous section, we denote by $(X_1, Y_1), (X_2, Y_2), \ldots, (X_n, Y_n)$ a sample of paired observations made on n individuals. We let $D_1 = X_1 - Y_1, D_2 = X_2 - Y_2, \ldots, D_n - X_n - Y_n$ be the corresponding differences. We assume that the differences $D_1, D_2, \ldots, D_n$ are normally distributed. We want to compare the average difference $\mu_D = \mu_X - \mu_Y$ with the value 0, by using a test of hypothesis. More precisely, we confront the null hypothesis $H_0 : \mu_D = 0$ with one of the alternatives $H_1 : \mu_D > 0$ or $H_1 : \mu_D < 0$.

By Theorem 9.4, if H_0 is true, then the test statistic

$$T_0 = \frac{\bar{D} - 0}{S_d/\sqrt{n}} \quad \text{has a } T(n-1) \text{ distribution.}$$

We consider separately the two cases:

Case (1) $H_0 : \mu_D = 0$ versus $H_1 : \mu_D > 0$

In this case, we want to reject H_0 and gain evidence that the average difference μ_D is positive, i.e. μ_X is larger than μ_Y. Our decision is based on the p-value. To perform the test, we calculate the observed value of the test statistic:

$$t_0 = \frac{\bar{d} - 0}{s_d/\sqrt{n}}. \tag{13.1}$$

If this (positive) ratio is large, then it is unlikely that H_0 is true, and there is some evidence in favor of H_1. The fact that the ratio is large corresponds to a small p-value, which is calculated as:

$$p\text{-value} = P(T > t_0),$$

where T is a random variable with a $T(n-1)$-distribution. If the p-value is small (usually smaller than 0.05), we reject H_0 and conclude that there is some evidence for H_1. Otherwise, we do not reject H_0.

Example 13.3. In the study [42], a group of 15 rats were inoculated in each hind leg with a $50\mu l$ injection of a colon tumor cell suspension (DHD/K12/TRb). The cell inoculation grew into a solid tumor at the injection site, which was used to model colon cancer. 6 weeks after the tumor inoculations, a drug called doxorubicin (Dox) was administered weekly to the rats. Each rat had one of the two tumors exposed to low-frequency ultrasound for an hour every week. At the end of the treatment time, the tumor volumes were measured in both legs. The table below gives for each rat the volume of the tumor in the leg which received only Dox (the x measurement) and the volume of the tumor in the leg which received Dox and ultrasound treatment (the y measurement). In all 15 rats, it was observed that the volume of the insonated (i.e. ultrasound treated) tumor is smaller than the volume of the noninsonated tumor.

Noninsonated Tumor (x_i)	Insonated Tumor (y_i)	Difference $d_i = x_i - y_i$
17.5	13.9	3.6
19.9	18.5	1.4
20.7	16.4	4.3
17.7	14.3	3.4
21.5	12.5	9.0
18.7	14.4	4.3
16.5	11.7	4.8
22.1	17.4	4.7
18.6	10.8	7.8
20.5	13.2	7.3
17.6	15.4	2.2
15.7	10.7	5.0
20.5	19.6	0.9
18.3	16.3	2.0
19.7	15.6	4.1

We assume that the difference data set has a normal distribution, an assumption which is supported by the QQ-plot.

We want to confront the hypothesis $H_0 : \mu_D = 0$ (which says that there is no difference between the volumes of the two tumors), with the alternative hypothesis $H_1 : \mu_D > 0$ (which says that noninsonated tumors have larger volumes, on average). The sample mean and the sample standard deviation of the (x, y) measurements are: $\bar{x} = 19.033$, $s_x = 1.858$, $\bar{y} = 14.713, s_y = 2.682$. These statistics are not needed for the analysis. What we need are the sample mean and the sample standard deviation of the differences: $\bar{d} = 4.32$ and $s_d = 2.318$.

The observed value of the test statistic is

$$t_0 = \frac{\bar{d} - 0}{s_d/\sqrt{n}} = \frac{4.32 - 0}{2.318/\sqrt{15}} = 7.218.$$

From Table 17.4, we see that $P(T > 2.997) = 0.005$ where T is a random variable with a $T(14)$ distribution. Since the observed value 7.218 is larger than 2.997, we infer that

$$p\text{-value} = P(T > 7.218) < 0.005.$$

The p-value being very small, we reject H_0 and conclude that the noninsonated tumors have larger volumes, on average, than the insonated tumors.

Case (2) $H_0 : \mu_D = 0$ versus $H_1 : \mu_D < 0$

In this case, we want to reject H_0 and gain evidence that the average difference μ_D is negative, i.e. μ_X is smaller than μ_Y. To perform the test, we calculate the same ratio t_0 given by (13.1) as in Case (1). If the absolute value of this (negative) ratio is large, then it is unlikely that H_0 is true, and there is some evidence in favor of H_1. The p-value is calculated as:

$$p\text{-value} = P(T < t_0),$$

where T is a random variable with a $T(n-1)$-distribution. If the p-value is small, we reject H_0 and conclude that there is some evidence for H_1. Otherwise, we do not reject H_0.

Example 13.4. Exercise therapy has been shown to influence human cartilage properties (see [4]). Shortly after exercise, it was noticed an elevation of serum levels of cartilage oligomeric matrix protein (COMP). The following table gives the serum COMP levels for 12 patients before 60 minutes of exercise (the x-measurement) and right after the exercise period (the y-measurement).

Before Exercise (x_i)	After Exercise (y_i)	Difference $d_i = x_i - y_i$
6.32	6.48	−0.16
7.85	8.27	−0.42
12.87	13.26	−0.39
11.27	11.84	−0.57
7.89	8.23	−0.34
15.56	15.87	−0.31
16.34	16.60	−0.26
7.83	8.17	−0.34
9.23	9.61	−0.38
10.22	10.38	−0.16
14.67	14.91	−0.24
15.30	15.61	−0.31

From this data, we notice an increase in the serum COMP levels due to the exercise. The assumption of normality of the differences appears to be verified. The sample means and sample standard deviations for the (x, y) measurements and the differences are given below:

	Before	After	Difference
Mean	$\bar{x} = 11.28$	$\bar{y} = 11.60$	$\bar{d} = -0.323$
Standard deviation	$s_x = 3.56$	$s_y = 3.55$	$s_d = 0.114$

We want to test $H_0 : \mu_D = 0$ against $H_1 : \mu_D < 0$. The observed value of the test statistic is

$$t_0 = \frac{\bar{d} - 0}{s_d/\sqrt{n}} = \frac{-0.323 - 0}{0.114/\sqrt{12}} = -9.82.$$

From Table 17.4, we see that $P(T < -3.106) = 0.005$ where T is a random variable with a $T(11)$ distribution. Since the observed value -9.82 is smaller than -3.106, we infer that

$$p\text{-value} = P(T < -9.82) < 0.005.$$

The p-value being very small, we reject H_0 and conclude that the serum COMP levels increase after exercise (on average).

13.3 Problems

Problem 13.1. Exposure to volatile organic compounds (VOC) which have been identified in indoor air is suspected as a cause for headaches and respiratory symptoms. Indoor plants have not only a positive psychological effects on humans, but may also improve the air quality. Certain species of indoor plants were found to be effective removers of VOCs. The following data gives the benzene level (in ppm) in 10 test chambers measured at the beginning of the study and after 3 days, using the plant *Epipremnum aureum* (Devils Ivy).

Initial Benzene Level (x_i)	Benzene level after 3 days (y_i)
28.4	27.4
27.3	26.3
25.5	25.6
29.4	24.5
30.2	28.7
31.3	29.6
28.6	27.5
28.4	28.4
26.5	23.2
27.3	24.3

Is there any evidence that this species of indoor plants is effective in removing the benzene from the indoor air? Justify your answer using a 95% confidence interval and a test of hypothesis. (Verify first that the differences $d_i = x_i - y_i, i = 1, \ldots, 10$ satisfy the normality assumption.)

Problem 13.2. The purpose of the study [29] was to determine whether twelve months of intense exercise training can induce an increase in left ventricular stroke volume in patients with coronary artery disease. 11 male patients were studied. Before training, the mean stroke volume was 66 ml/beat and the standard deviation 11 ml/beat. After training, the mean stroke volume was 81 ml/beat and the standard deviation 13 ml/beat. The standard deviation of the differences between the stroke volume before the exercise program and after the program was 5.4 ml/beat. Do these findings suggest that prolonged and intense training induces an increase in stroke volume in patients with coronary artery disease ? Justify your answer using a 95% confidence interval for the mean difference between the stroke volume before the exercising program, and after the program.

Problem 13.3. Almost two-thirds of iron in the body is found in hemoglobin, the protein in the red blood cells that carries oxygen to the tissues. Iron deficiency could lead to anemia, a condition characterized by less than the normal quantity of hemoglobin in the blood. The following data gives the hemoglobin values for 7 female patients at risk for anemia, before and after they followed a 3-month dietary iron intake program:

Before	After
10.4	12.3
11.5	13.6
9.6	13.7
8.7	10.3
11.5	14.3
11.8	13.9
10.7	12.8

(a) Was the program efficient in increasing the hemoglobin level? Justify your answer using a test of hypothesis for $H_0 : \mu_1 = \mu_2$ against $H_1 : \mu_1 < \mu_2$, where μ_1 and μ_2 are the average hemoglobin levels before, respectively after the program. Use the level $\alpha = 0.005$.
(b) What is the conclusion of a test of level $\alpha = 0.005$, if we assume (incorrectly) that the hemoglobin level after the program is independent of the hemoglobin level before the program? Assume that the two populations are normally distributed with equal variances.

Problem 13.4. Two different methods were used to measure the cisternal milk volume (in kg) for 10 cows.

Cow	Method 1	Method 2
1	1.39	1.46
2	1.54	1.56
3	1.62	1.61
4	1.70	1.74
5	1.71	1.76
6	1.73	1.76
7	1.73	1.84
8	1.81	1.90
9	1.85	1.95
10	1.91	2.02

Do the methods give significantly different measurements on average? Use the significance level $\alpha = 0.05$.

Problem 13.5. An experiment was designed to test the effects of a growth hormone (GH) on the daily milk production. The study involved ten pairs of identical twin dairy cows. For each pair of twins, only one cow was given the growth hormone, the other being considered a control. The table below gives the milk production (in kg per day) for each set of twins.

Twin set	Control	GH
1	9.86	9.69
2	12.10	12.38
3	13.33	14.24
4	13.69	14.09
5	9.04	9.05
6	9.72	10.67
7	9.89	11.48
8	10.22	11.14
9	9.46	9.54
10	9.02	9.05

Is there any evidence that the growth hormone increases the milk production? Justify your answer using a 98% confidence interval and a test of hypothesis at level $\alpha = 0.025$. (Verify first that the normality assumption is satisfied.)

Problem 13.6. We wish to compare the effect of two preparations of a virus on tobacco plants. The study involves 8 plants. For each plant, half a leaf is inoculated with preparation 1 and the other half is inoculated with preparation 2. The number of lesions are measured and denoted as x_1 and x_2, respectively. The data are given in the following table.

plant	x_1	x_2	plant	x_1	x_2
1	30	20	11	18	16
2	8	5	12	14	13
3	14	17	13	12	4
4	14	11	14	13	13
5	19	17	15	16	14
6	17	15	16	16	14
7	3	5	17	18	12
8	19	15	18	21	15
9	12	12	19	12	10
10	21	14	20	17	12

(a) Do the preparations have a different effect on the tobacco plants? Justify your answer using a test of hypothesis for $H_0 : \mu_1 = \mu_2$ against $H_1 : \mu_1 \neq \mu_2$, where μ_1 is the mean number of lesions when preparation 1 is used and μ_2 is the mean number of lesions when preparation 2 is used. Use the level $\alpha = 0.05$.
(b) What is the conclusion of a test of level $\alpha = 0.05$, if we assume (incorrectly) that the observations from the same plant are independent? Assume that the two populations are normally distributed with equal variances.

Problem 13.7. An new surgical procedure is compared to the old method. Fifteen surgeons perform the operation on two patients, who are similar in terms of relevant factors such as age and gender. The table below gives the duration (in minutes) for each surgery.

surgeon	Old Method	New Method	surgeon	Old Method	New Method
1	33.1	31.4	9	19.9	21.7
2	46.6	40.5	10	46.0	36.6
3	21.5	29.9	11	49.0	54.7
4	34.3	45.0	12	45.5	39.5
5	19.1	12.5	13	60.3	61.2
6	38.9	44.0	14	37.4	34.0
7	56.2	57.2	15	25.3	19.1
8	67.1	65.6			

Is there any evidence that the new surgical procedure will reduce the duration of the surgery? Justify your answer with a test of hypothesis at level $\alpha = 0.05$. (Verify first that the normality assumption is satisfied.)

Did you know that? *Haemophilia is a rare hereditary disease, characterized by an impaired ability of blood coagulation. Bleeding is a general symptom of the disease, but one of the difficulties in recognizing the presence of the disease is that bleeding can be internal. The disease is more likely to occur in males, but females can transmit it to their offsprings. Haemophilia is sometimes called "the royal disease", since it occurred frequently among the European royal families. It is thought that Queen Victoria inherited the gene and passed the mutation through her children, across the European continent, to the royal families of Spain, Germany, and Russia. Alexei Nikolaevich, the only son of Russia's last tsar Nicholas II, was a descendant of Queen Victoria through his mother Empress Alexandra, and suffered from haemophilia. According to some sources, the mystic healer Rasputin succeeded in treating the son's tsar, by simply advising against the traditional medical treatment with aspirin.*

Chapter 14

Categorical Data

In this chapter, we consider two categorical variables X and Y, i.e. variables whose values may not be numeric, but can be classified in several classes. Examples of such variables include: gender, blood type, age, race, income level, home ownership status, level of education, etc. Using the method of hypothesis testing, the goal is to gain evidence that there is an association between X and Y. This is called a test of independence. We also discuss the test of homogeneity, for which we examine several groups which underwent distinct treatments whose results are classified using a categorical variable X. In this case, we want to gain evidence that there is a significant difference between the groups, from the point of view of the proportion of individuals falling in the classes of the variable X.

14.1 Test of Independence

In this section, we investigate if there is an association between two categorical variables X and Y. We assume that X has r classes, and Y has c classes. Every individual in the sample is classified according to both X and Y, and falls precisely into one class for each variable. For instance, if X is the gender, and Y is the smoking status, then X has $r = 2$ classes (male, female), Y has $c = 2$ classes (smoker, non-smoker), and each individual is classified into one of the 4 possible categories (or cells): smoker male, smoker female, non-smoker male, non-smoker female.

Our goal is to gain evidence that there is a relationship between X and Y. Keeping in mind that we aim to reject H_0, we let:

$$H_0: \text{ } X \text{ and } Y \text{ are independent}$$
$$H_1: \text{ there is an association between } X \text{ and } Y.$$

This is called a *test of independence.*

Example 14.1. The purpose of the study [28] was to identify some eating and physical activity patterns associated with overweight elementary school children in Fort Worth, Texas, by comparison with the guidelines of the United States Department of Agriculture and the National Association for Sports and Physical Activities. The 1,018 participant children were classified according to various criteria. In particular, they were classified according to race (variable X), as 571 Hispanic and 447 African American. These numbers were random, i.e. they were not fixed by the researchers at the beginning of the study. The children were also classified according to weight (variable Y): in the group of Hispanic children, 105 were overweight or at risk of being overweight, whereas in the group of African American children, 208 were overweight or at risk of being overweight. The data is summarized in the table below:

	normal weight	overweight	Total
Hispanic	466	105	571 (random)
African American	239	208	447 (random)
Total	705 (random)	313 (random)	1,018

Based on this data, we want to see if there is an association between the race and the risk of being overweight, for the children in this Texas community.

Example 14.2. The distribution of the blood type in a population is known to be different in each continent: for instance, the proportion of people with type B blood is significantly different in Asia and Europe. Despite this fact, matching personality traits with one's blood type is a popular phenomenon in Japan and South Korea (similar to the horoscope matching with personality, in the Western countries), whose scientific grounds are still debatable. In the following table, 100 individuals of Asian descent were classified according to their predominant personality trait (the variable X) and their blood group (the variable Y) in 8 classes. Note that the row totals and the column totals are random, i.e. they could not be predicted by the researcher at the beginning of the experiment.

	O	A	B	AB	Total
Artistic	17	15	14	2	48
Practical	23	11	13	5	52
Total	40	26	27	7	100

Based on this data, we want to see if there is an association between the personality and the blood type, for the people of Asian descent.

To illustrate the general theory, we denote by n_{ij} the number of observations (or frequencies) corresponding to class i of variable X and class j of variable Y, for $i = 1, 2, \ldots, r$ and $j = 1, 2, \ldots, c$. Thus n_{ij} is the number of individuals in the sample, who fall in the (i, j)-category. The frequencies corresponding to the $r \times c$ categories (or cells) are displayed in a *contingency table*:

	Class B_1	Class B_2	......	Class B_c	Total
Class A_1	n_{11}	n_{12}	......	n_{1c}	$n_{1\cdot}$
Class A_2	n_{21}	n_{22}	......	n_{2c}	$n_{2\cdot}$
...	...	...	......	...	...
Class A_r	n_{r1}	n_{r2}	......	n_{rc}	$n_{r\cdot}$
Total	$n_{\cdot 1}$	$n_{\cdot 2}$	......	$n_{\cdot c}$	n

We calculate the totals for each row and for each column:

$n_{i\cdot} = n_{i1} + n_{i2} + \cdots + n_{ic}$ is the total for row i, with $i = 1, 2, \ldots, r$

$n_{\cdot j} = n_{1j} + n_{2j} + \cdots + n_{rj}$ is the total for column j, with $j = 1, 2, \ldots, c$.

Then the total number of observations is:

$$\begin{aligned} n &= n_{1\cdot} + n_{2\cdot} + \cdots + n_{r\cdot} \quad \text{(the sum of row totals)} \\ &= n_{\cdot 1} + n_{\cdot 2} + \cdots + n_{\cdot c} \quad \text{(the sum of column totals).} \end{aligned}$$

To perform a test of independence, it is important to make sure that all the row totals and column totals are random, i.e. none of these totals is known to the researcher, prior to the experiment. We rephrase hypothesis H_0 in a more convenient form. Recall from Chapter 5 that two events A and B are independent if

$$P(A \cap B) = P(A)P(B).$$

We denote by p_{ij} the probability that a random observation falls into the (i, j)-cell of the table (i.e. row i, column j). We let $p_{i\cdot}$ be the probability that a random observation falls in row i, and $p_{\cdot j}$ the probability that a random observation falls in column j. Hypothesis H_0 can be restated as:

$$H_0 : p_{ij} = p_{i\cdot} p_{\cdot j} \quad \text{for every } i \text{ and for every } j.$$

Estimators for the probabilities $p_{i\cdot}$ and $p_{\cdot j}$ are, respectively:

$$\hat{p}_{i\cdot} = \frac{n_{i\cdot}}{n}, \quad \hat{p}_{\cdot j} = \frac{n_{\cdot j}}{n}.$$

If H_0 is true, then $\hat{p}_{ij} = \hat{p}_{i\cdot}\hat{p}_{\cdot j}$ is an estimator for p_{ij}. In this case, the "expected" number of observations falling into the (i, j)-cell is:

$$\hat{E}_{ij} = n\hat{p}_{ij} = n\hat{p}_{i\cdot}\hat{p}_{\cdot j} = n\left(\frac{n_{i\cdot}}{n}\right)\left(\frac{n_{\cdot j}}{n}\right) = \frac{n_{i\cdot}n_{\cdot j}}{n}.$$

This number may be different from the observed number n_{ij} of observations in the (i, j)-cell. If so, then there is some evidence that hypothesis H_0 is not true. But how different should $\hat{E}_{ij}$ be from n_{ij}, in order to reject H_0?

To answer this question, we note first that our conclusion has to be based on all the observations, not only on those falling into one particular cell. Therefore, we calculate all the differences $n_{ij} - \hat{E}_{ij}$, hoping that the majority of them are large positive numbers, in absolute value. Secondly, we square these differences so that the negative values are not counterbalanced by the positive ones. Finally, these differences have to be properly normalized to obtain a random variable which has a known distribution. Using methods which are beyond the scope of this book, it can be proved that the test statistic:

$$U_0 = \sum_{i=1}^{r}\sum_{j=1}^{c}\frac{(n_{ij} - \hat{E}_{ij})^2}{\hat{E}_{ij}} \quad \text{has a } \chi^2\text{-distribution.}$$

The χ^2-distribution is an asymmetric distribution, which depends on one parameter, called "the number of degrees of freedom". In the case of the variable above, the number of degrees of freedom is $(r - 1)(c - 1)$. Probabilities associated with χ^2 random variables are given in Table 17.5.

A large value of the sum of the normalized square differences (given by the observed value u_0 of the test statistic U_0) is an indication that H_0 is not true. To decide if this value u_0 is large enough, compared with values that may arise from other samples, we calculate the following:

$$p\text{-value} = P(U > u_0),$$

where U is a random variable with a χ^2 distribution with $(r - 1)(c - 1)$ degrees of freedom. The smaller the p-value, the less likely it is that H_0 is true.

If a preset α-level is specified for the probability of the type I error, then we reject H_0 when the p-value is smaller than α. In this case, we say that there is some evidence for an association between X and Y. On the other hand, if the p-value is larger than α, we fail to reject H_0. In this case, we do not have enough evidence that there is an association between X and Y.

Example 14.1 (Continued). We set up the following hypotheses:

H_0 : race and risk of being overweight are independent

H_1 : there is an association between the race and the risk of being overweight.

We calculate the "expected" number of observations for each cell:

$$\hat{E}_{11} = \frac{571 \cdot 705}{1018} = 395.44, \quad \hat{E}_{12} = \frac{571 \cdot 313}{1018} = 175.56,$$
$$\hat{E}_{21} = \frac{447 \cdot 705}{1018} = 309.56, \quad \hat{E}_{22} = \frac{447 \cdot 313}{1018} = 137.44.$$

We put these values in the table underneath the observed values, in parenthesis:

	normal weight	overweight	Total
Hispanic	466 (395.44)	105 (175.56)	571
African American	239 (309.56)	208 (137.44)	447
Total	705	313	1018

The observed value of the test statistic is:

$$u_0 = \frac{(466 - 395.44)^2}{395.44} + \frac{(105 - 175.56)^2}{175.56} + \frac{(239 - 309.56)^2}{309.56}$$
$$+ \frac{(208 - 137.44)^2}{137.44} = 93.265$$

Then, p-value $= P(U > 93.265)$, where U is a random variable with a χ^2 distribution with $(2-1)(2-1) = 1$ degree of freedom. For this distribution, the last value that we read in Table 17.5 is 7.879, i.e. $P(U > 7.879) = 0.005$. Hence,

$$p\text{-value} < 0.005.$$

Since the p-value is very small, we conclude that there is enough evidence in this data to support the claim that there is an association between the race and the risk of being overweight, for the children in this community.

Example 14.2 (Continued). We set up the following hypotheses:

H_0 : personality and blood type are independent

H_1 : there is an association between personality and blood type.

We calculate the "expected" number of observations for each cell:

$$\hat{E}_{11} = \frac{48 \cdot 40}{100} = 19.20, \quad \hat{E}_{12} = \frac{48 \cdot 26}{100} = 12.48,$$
$$\hat{E}_{13} = \frac{48 \cdot 27}{100} = 12.96, \quad \hat{E}_{14} = \frac{48 \cdot 7}{100} = 3.36,$$
$$\hat{E}_{21} = \frac{52 \cdot 40}{100} = 20.80, \quad \hat{E}_{22} = \frac{52 \cdot 26}{100} = 13.52,$$
$$\hat{E}_{23} = \frac{52 \cdot 27}{100} = 14.04, \quad \hat{E}_{24} = \frac{52 \cdot 7}{100} = 3.64.$$

We put these values in the table underneath the observed values, in parenthesis:

	O	A	B	AB	Total
Artistic	17 (19.20)	15 (12.48)	14 (12.96)	2 (3.36)	48
Practical	23 (20.80)	11 (13.52)	13 (14.04)	5 (3.64)	52
Total	40	26	27	7	100

The observed value of the test statistic is:

$$u_0 = \frac{(17-19.2)^2}{19.2} + \frac{(15-12.48)^2}{12.48} + \frac{(14-12.96)^2}{12.96} + \frac{(2-3.36)^2}{3.36}$$
$$+ \frac{(23-20.8)^2}{20.8} + \frac{(11-13.52)^2}{13.52} + \frac{(13-14.04)^2}{14.04} + \frac{(5-3.64)^2}{3.64} = 2.682.$$

Then, p-value $= P(U > 2.682)$, where U is a random variable with a χ^2 distribution with $(2-1)(4-1) = 3$ degrees of freedom. Looking on row 3 of Table 17.5, we see that 2.682 lies between 2.366 (whose corresponding area to right is 0.50) and 4.108 (whose corresponding area to right is 0.25). We conclude that:

$$0.25 < p\text{-value} < 0.50.$$

Using a statistical software, we see that p-value$= 0.443$. Since the p-value is very large, this data does not support the claim that there in an association between personality and blood type, for people of Asian descent.

14.2 Test of Homogeneity

In this section, we consider r experimental groups which are classified in several classes according to a categorical variable X. The size of each group is fixed, and is decided by the researcher at the beginning of the study. We want to gain evidence that the groups are significantly different, from the point of view of this classification. More precisely, we want to show that the proportions of items falling into the same classification class are different among the r groups. For instance, four groups of plants are treated with different fertilizers, and their growth after one month is classified as low, average or high. We want to show that there is a difference between these four groups, in the sense that we observe a difference between the proportions of plants with low growth, average growth, or high growth among the four groups.

Example 14.3. Human Papillomavirus (HPV) can infect different parts of the body. Most HPV infections occur without any symptoms and go away without treatment over the course of a few years. However, in some people, HPV infections can persist. This is especially dangerous if the persistent infection is of a cancer-causing type. Persistent HPV infection of a cancer-causing type is the major cause of cervical cancer. Gardasil is a vaccine which is designed to prevent infection with HPV types 6, 11, 16 and 18, and was approved by Health Canada in July 2006, for use among girls and women 9 to 26 years old. 10,565 women between the ages of 15 and 26 participated in a large clinical study, whose results were published in [24]. These women received three doses of either HPV-6/11/16/18 vaccine or placebo, administered at day 1, month 2 and month 6. These subjects were followed for an average of 3 years after receiving the first dose of vaccine or placebo. Among the 5,305 women who received the vaccine, 1 was diagnosed with cervical cancer. In the group of 5,260 women who received the placebo, 42 were diagnosed with cervical cancer. The results are summarized in the table below:

	cervical cancer: yes	cervical cancer: no	Total
Group 1: vaccine	1	5,304	5,305 (fixed)
Group 2: placebo	42	5,218	5,260 (fixed)
Total	43	10,522	10,565

We want to gain evidence for the hypothesis that the proportions of women with cervical cancer are not the same in the two groups.

Example 14.4. The Forest Stewardship Council (FSC) is an international, membership-based, non-profit organization that supports environmentally appropriate, socially beneficial, and economically viable management of the world's forests. The FSC was founded in 1993 in Toronto, Canada by representatives from environmental groups, the timber industry, the forestry profession, and community groups from 26 countries. In 2008, there were over 100 million hectares in more than 80 countries certified according to FSC standards. Since consumers are increasingly concerned about the impact of their decisions on the environment, there is a growing number of companies which are using FSC-certified products. In the table below, a sample of 100 companies were given a reputation score (between A and E) based on the customer satisfaction, quality of products, media and public relation, and international recognition. 50 of these companies use FSC-certified products, whereas the other 50 do not.

	A	B	C	D	E	Total
Use FSC products	8	13	16	10	3	50 (fixed)
Do not use FSC products	4	9	14	16	7	50 (fixed)
Total	12	22	30	26	10	100

We want to get evidence that there is a difference between the companies which use FSC products and the companies which do not use them, from the point of view of their reputation.

To illustrate the general theory, we suppose that the r groups are classified according to a categorical variable which has c classes. We denote by n_{ij} the number of observations in the i-th group, which fall in the j-th class. We organize the information as in Section 14.1 in a *contingency table*:

	Class 1	Class 2	......	Class c	Total
Group 1	n_{11}	n_{12}	......	n_{1c}	$n_{1\cdot}$ (fixed)
Group 2	n_{21}	n_{22}	......	n_{2c}	$n_{2\cdot}$ (fixed)
...	...	...	......	...	...
Group r	n_{r1}	n_{r2}	......	n_{rc}	$n_{r\cdot}$ (fixed)
Total	$n_{\cdot 1}$	$n_{\cdot 2}$	......	$n_{\cdot c}$	n

We calculate the following totals:

$$n_{i\cdot} = \sum_{j=1}^{c} n_{ij} \quad \text{is the total number of observations in the } i\text{-th group,}$$

$$n_{\cdot j} = \sum_{i=1}^{r} n_{ij} \quad \text{is the total number of observations in the } j\text{-th class.}$$

The total number of observations is:

$$\begin{aligned} n &= n_{1\cdot} + n_{2\cdot} + \ldots + n_r \\ &= n_{\cdot 1} + n_{\cdot 2} + \ldots + n_{\cdot c}. \end{aligned}$$

Let p_{ij} be the proportion of individuals in the i-th group, who fall in the j-th class. We want to gain evidence that the proportions p_{ij} are not all the same in the r groups. Keeping in mind that our goal is to reject H_0, we set up the following hypotheses:

H_0 : $p_{1j} = p_{2j} = \ldots = p_{rj}$, for all $j = 1, 2, \ldots, c$.

H_1 : the proportions $p_{1j}, p_{2j}, \ldots, p_{rj}$ are not the same, for at least one j.

This is called a *test of homogeneity.*

Note that p_{ij} can be interpreted as the conditional probability that an individual falls in the j-th category, given that he or she belongs to the i-th group. Hypothesis H_0 says that for every category, these conditional probabilities are the same for the r groups.

If H_0 is true, an estimate for the common value $p_j := p_{1j} = p_{2j} = \ldots = p_{rj}$ is:

$$\hat{p}_j = \frac{n_{\cdot j}}{n}.$$

This is an estimate for the proportion of individuals of the i-th group, falling in the j-th class. Since the i-th group has size $n_{i\cdot}$, the expected number of individuals from the i-th group, falling in the j-th class is (if H_0 is true):

$$\hat{E}_{ij} = n_{i\cdot}\hat{p}_j = \frac{n_{i\cdot}n_{\cdot j}}{n}.$$

(Note that this coincides with the expected number of observations in the case of a test of independence. The interpretation is different this time.)

The number $\hat{E}_{ij}$, which we expect to observe if H_0 is true, has to be compared with the observed number n_{ij}. A large difference (in absolute value) between $\hat{E}_{ij}$ and n_{ij} is an indication that H_0 is not true. To see if n_{ij} deviates significantly from $\hat{E}_{ij}$ throughout the table, we calculate the sum of the normalized squared differences $(\hat{E}_{ij} - n_{ij})^2/\hat{E}_{ij}$. As in Section 14.1, we use the fact that the test statistic:

$$U_0 = \sum_{i=1}^{r}\sum_{j=1}^{c} \frac{(\hat{E}_{ij} - n_{ij})^2}{\hat{E}_{ij}} \quad \text{has a } \chi^2\text{-distribution}$$

with $(r-1)(c-1)$ degrees of freedom. A large observed value u_0 of this test statistic is strong evidence against H_0. To decide if this sum if large enough for rejecting H_0, we calculate:

$$p\text{-value} = P(U > u_0),$$

where U is a random variable with a χ^2 distribution with $(r-1)(c-1)$ degrees of freedom.

Example 14.3 (Continued). We set up the following hypotheses:

H_0 : the proportions of cervical cancer in the two groups are the same

H_1 : the proportions of cervical cancer in the two groups are different.

We calculate the "expected" number of observations for each cell:

$$\hat{E}_{11} = \frac{5305 \cdot 43}{10565} = 21.59, \quad \hat{E}_{12} = \frac{5305 \cdot 10522}{10565} = 5283.41,$$
$$\hat{E}_{21} = \frac{5260 \cdot 43}{10565} = 21.41, \quad \hat{E}_{22} = \frac{5260 \cdot 10522}{10565} = 5238.60.$$

The observed value of the test statistic is:

$$u_0 = \frac{(1-21.59)^2}{21.59} + \frac{(5304-5283.41)^2}{5283.41} + \frac{(42-21.41)^2}{21.41} + \frac{(5218-5238.60)^2}{5238.60} = 39.60.$$

Using Table 17.5, we infer that:

$$p\text{-value} = P(U > 39.60) < 0.005,$$

where U is a random variable with a χ^2-distribution with $(2-1)(2-1) = 1$ degree of freedom. Since the p-value is very small, we reject H_0. We conclude that there is enough evidence that the proportions of cervical cancer are different in the two groups.

Example 14.4 (Continued). We set up the following hypotheses:

H_0 : the proportions of companies who received any given score (between A and F) are the same in the two groups

H_1 : there is at least one score (between A and F) for which the proportions of companies are different in the two groups.

We calculate the "expected" numbers for each cell:

$$\hat{E}_{11} = \hat{E}_{21} = \frac{50 \cdot 12}{100} = 6, \quad \hat{E}_{12} = \hat{E}_{22} = \frac{50 \cdot 22}{100} = 11$$
$$\hat{E}_{13} = \hat{E}_{23} = \frac{50 \cdot 30}{100} = 15, \quad \hat{E}_{14} = \hat{E}_{24} = \frac{50 \cdot 26}{100} = 13$$
$$\hat{E}_{15} = \hat{E}_{25} = \frac{50 \cdot 10}{100} = 5.$$

Because the sample sizes are the same for the two groups, the values on the first row are identical with the values on the second row. The observed value of the test statistic is:

$$u_0 = \frac{(8-6)^2}{6} + \frac{(13-11)^2}{11} + \frac{(16-15)^2}{15} + \frac{(10-13)^2}{13} + \frac{(3-5)^2}{5}$$

$$+\frac{(4-6)^2}{6} + \frac{(9-11)^2}{11} + \frac{(14-15)^2}{15} + \frac{(16-13)^2}{13} + \frac{(7-5)^2}{5} = 5.179.$$

Then, p-value $= P(U > 4.38)$, where U is a random variable with a χ^2 distribution with $(2-1)(5-1) = 4$ degrees of freedom. Using Table 17.5, we conclude that:

$$0.25 < p\text{-value} < 0.5.$$

Using a statistical software, we see that p-value$= 0.269$. Since the p-value is large, we fail to reject H_0. We conclude that the two groups of companies do not differ significantly from the point of view of customer rating.

14.3 Problems

Problem 14.1. Lung cancers are classified using the size and appearance of the malignant cells as seen by a histopathologist under a microscope as: non-small cell lung carcinoma or small cell lung carcinoma. The non-small cell lung carcinomas are the most frequently encountered types of lung cancer, and are divided into three sub-types: squamous cell lung carcinoma, adenocarcinoma, and large cell lung carcinoma. Using the data given in the table below, can we conclude that the proportions of the three sub-types of non-small cell lung carcinomas are different in the smoker population and the non-smoker population?

	Squamous cell lung carcinoma	Adenocarcinoma	Large cell lung carcinoma
Smokers	42	43	15
Non-smokers	33	45	22

Problem 14.2. To test the claim that nitrogen trichloride (produced by chlorine) is a cause of occupational asthma in indoor swimming pool workers, a group of 625 lifeguards and swim instructors were asked to fill out a questionnaire regarding respiratory symptoms and the number of hours spent in the facility per week. The data is presented in the following table:

Number of hours	Respiratory Symptoms None	Mild	Severe	Total
less than 12	256	34	24	314
12 to 19	159	26	20	205
20 to 32	45	8	10	63
more than 32	29	6	8	43
Total	489	74	62	625

Is there enough evidence that there is an association between the respiratory symptoms and the number of hours spent in the swimming pool for the swimming pool workers?

Problem 14.3. In the developed countries, one of the factors leading to child obesity could be the family income. It is estimated that in Canada, the national combined overweight/obesity rate for children and adolescents of ages 2 to 17 is 33%. The following table gives the data obtained for 1,570 children, who were classified according to weight and annual family income:

Annual Family Income	Weight Normal	Overweight/obese	Total
under \$40,000	95	65	160
\$40,000-\$80,000	412	278	690
\$80,000-\$120,000	322	188	510
over \$120,000	151	59	210
Total	980	590	1570

Can we conclude that there is an association between the family income and the child's weight? Use the significance level $\alpha = 0.05$.

Problem 14.4. The authors of [1] studied human-bear interactions in Delani National Park (United States). The following table summarizes 192 human-bear interactions by giving the conditional relative frequency distributions of bear behaviour according to the type of area. The sample sizes corresponding to "in developed areas", "in camp", "on park road" and "in the back-country" are 17, 50, 42 and 83, respectively.

Type of Area	Behaviour Displayed			
	Aggression	Approach	Neutral	Avoidance
Developed Areas	6%	70%	12%	12%
In Camp	2%	64%	20%	14%
On Park Road	17%	40%	12%	31%
Back-Country	6%	25 %	6%	63%

Can we conclude that there is an association between the behaviour displayed and the type of area? Use the significance level $\alpha = 0.05$. Hint: Calculate first the observed frequencies for each cell, by rounding to the closest integer.

Problem 14.5. Consider the germination data from Example 4.2. The data represents a random sample of 105 species that are cross-classified according to the germinability and the germination speed.

Germination Speed	Germinability			Total
	Low	Intermediate	High	
Fast	14	4	4	22
Medium	36	22	2	60
Slow	6	13	4	23
Total	56	39	10	105

Can we conclude that there is an association between the germinability and the germination speed? Use the significance level $\alpha = 0.05$.

Problem 14.6. The authors of [5] studied the behaviour of male adolescent smokeless tobacco users. Among 137 fathers, 70 reported using either smokeless tobacco or cigarettes. Among the fathers who use smokeless tobacco or cigarettes, 30% reported having sons who use smokeless tobacco daily. For the non-using fathers, only 10.4% reported having sons who use smokeless tobacco daily.

(a) Fill-out the following contingency table.

Father consumes tobacco	Have sons who use smokeless tobacco daily		Total
	Yes	No	
Yes			
No			
Total			

(b) Can we conclude that there is an association between the fathers' use of tobacco and the sons' daily use of smokeless tobacco? Use the significance level $\alpha = 0.05$.

Problem 14.7. The study [9] examined the flowering patterns of trees in a wet tropical forest. Some species of trees have flowers only in one wet season, others have flowers in both wet seasons, and others have flowers only in the dry season. The table below gives the frequency distribution of the flowering time for 7 families of trees. For instance, among the 11 observed species in the annonaceae family, 8 have flowers only in one wet season, 3 have flowers in both wet seasons, and 1 has flowers only in the dry season.

	Flowering Time		
Phylogeny	Only in one wet season	In both wet seasons	Only in dry season
Annonaceae	8	3	1
Euphorbiaceae	12	6	1
Lauraceae	9	1	4
Leguminosea	20	6	4
Moraceae	9	5	3
Palmae	15	4	2
Rubiaceae	16	5	5

Are the distributions of flowering time homogeneous across tree families? Assume that the observed numbers of species per family are fixed. Use the significance level $\alpha = 0.05$.

Did you know that? *Blood transfusions have been attempted for centuries to save patients' lives, with mixed results: occasionally the patient recovered, but often the patient died almost at once. This mystery was solved in 1901 by an Austrian biologist and physician, named Karl Landsteiner. By mixing red blood corpuscles from the blood of one individual with the serum from the blood of another, he identified the presence of agglutinin in the blood. For his discovery which led to the development of the modern system of classification of blood groups, Landsteiner received the Nobel Prize for Medicine in 1930. In 1946, together with Alexander Wiener and Philip Levine, he was awarded (posthumously) the Albert Lasker Award, for the discovery of the Rh factor and its significance as a cause of prenatal mortality.*

Chapter 15

Regression and Correlation

Biologists are often interested in the relationship between two variables. We learn in this chapter to describe the relationship between two quantitative variables with a line. This is called a regression analysis. We discuss inferences concerning a population regression line and we present tools to assess the validity of the underlying assumptions of the regression. We will learn to use the regression model to predict future values of one variable given a value of the other variable. We end with a discussion of correlation analysis. The correlation is a measure of the degree of association between two quantitative variables and is closely related to the regression analysis.

15.1 Least Squares Line

In this section, we begin by describing the association between a variable y (also called the *response*) and a variable x (also called the *predictor*) with a line of best fit. We assume that we have a random sample of paired observations (x_i, y_i) for $i = 1, \ldots, n$.

Example 15.1 (Part 1). Consider the data from Example 9.8. The predictor variable x is the dosage of vitamin C and the response variable y is the number of colds. For these data, the line of best fit is $\hat{y} = 12.0 - 0.0944\,x$, which is overlayed in the scatter plot in Figure 15.1.

To find the line of best fit, denoted by $\hat{y} = \hat{\alpha} + \hat{\beta}\,x$, we will define what we mean by "best". Consider the ith case (x_i, y_i). The corresponding *fitted value* $\hat{y}_i = \hat{\alpha} + \hat{\beta}\,x_i$ is the evaluation of the estimated line at $x = x_i$. The difference between the ith observed response and the ith fitted value is called the ith *residual* $e_i = y_i - \hat{y}_i$. A residual is sometimes called an

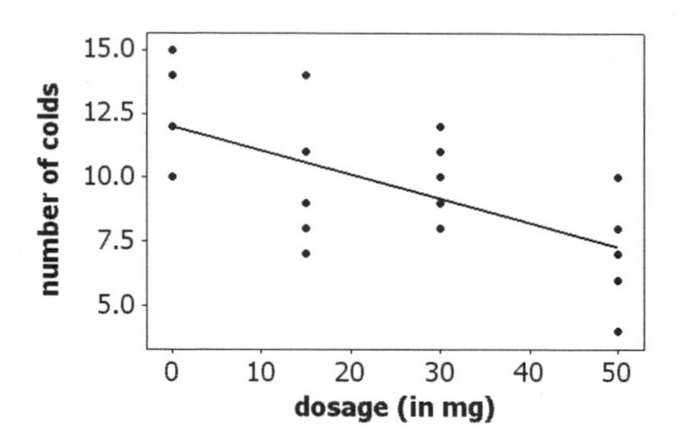

Fig. 15.1 Least squares line for the number of colds against dosage of vitamin C

observed error. The sum of the squared residuals:

$$L = \sum_{i=1}^{n} \left[y_i - (\hat{\alpha} + \hat{\beta}\, x_i) \right]^2,$$

is used as measure of fit. In some sense, L represents a distance between the observed responses and the estimated line. We say that the line of best fit is the line that minimizes L. This criterion of fit was independently proposed in the 18th century by the German mathematician Carl Friedrich Gauss and by the French mathematician Adrien-Marie Legendre. It is known as the *method of least-squares.*

The minimum of the least-squares criterion L can be found by differentiating it with respect to $\hat{\alpha}$ and $\hat{\beta}$ and by setting these partial derivatives equal to zero. We obtain a system of two equations in $\hat{\alpha}$ and $\hat{\beta}$ that we need to solve. After some simplification, these equations can be shown to be

$$\sum_{i=1}^{n} y_i = n\,\hat{\alpha} + \hat{\beta} \sum_{i=1}^{n} x_i \quad \text{and} \quad \sum_{i=1}^{n} x_i y_i = \hat{\alpha} \sum_{i=1}^{n} x_i + \hat{\beta} \sum_{i=1}^{n} x_i^2. \qquad (15.1)$$

These equations are called the *normal equations.* As we isolate $\hat{\alpha}$ in the first equation and substitute it in the second equation to obtain $\hat{\beta}$, we get the least-squares estimates of the intercept

$$\hat{\alpha} = \frac{\sum_{i=1}^{n} y_i}{n} - \hat{\beta}\, \frac{\sum_{i=1}^{n} x_i}{n}, \qquad (15.2)$$

and of the slope

$$\hat{\beta} = \frac{(\sum_{i=1}^n x_i\,y_i) - (1/n)(\sum_{i=1}^n x_i)(\sum_{i=1}^n y_i)}{(\sum_{i=1}^n x_i^2) - (1/n)(\sum_{i=1}^n x_i)^2} = \frac{\sum_{i=1}^n (x_i - \overline{x})(y_i - \overline{y})}{\sum_{i=1}^n (x_i - \overline{x})^2} = \frac{\sum_{i=1}^n (x_i - \overline{x})\,y_i}{(n-1)\,s_x^2}. \tag{15.3}$$

All the quantities involved in this solution should seem familiar. Actually the slope and the intercept of the least-squares line have a few other useful representations, such as

$$\hat{\beta} = \frac{\sum_{i=1}^n (x_i - \overline{x})(y_i - \overline{y})/(n-1)}{\sum_{i=1}^n (x_i - \overline{x})^2/(n-1)} = \frac{s_{xy}}{s_x^2} = r_{xy}\,\frac{s_y}{s_x}$$

and

$$\hat{\alpha} = \overline{y} - \hat{\beta}\,\overline{x} = \frac{1}{n}\sum_{i=1}^n y_i - \left(\frac{\sum_{i=1}^n (x_i - \overline{x})\,y_i}{(n-1)s_x^2}\right)\overline{x} = \sum_{i=1}^n \left[\frac{1}{n} - \frac{(x_i - \overline{x})\,\overline{x}}{(n-1)s_x^2}\right] y_i$$

where $\overline{x}$ and $\overline{y}$ are respectively the sample means of the predictors and the responses, s_x^2 is the sample variance of the predictors, s_{xy} is the sample covariance between x and y, and r_{xy} is the sample correlation between x and y. Recall that we defined these descriptive statistics in Section 9.1. Note that the slope of the least-squares line will always have the same sign as the sample correlation between the response and the predictor.

Some other properties of the least squares line can be derived from the normal equations. The line always passes through the centroid $(\overline{x}, \overline{y})$ of the sample. From the first normal equation, we can show that $\sum_{i=1}^n e_i = 0$. So the average of the residuals is equal to zero. The latter property also implies that $(1/n)\sum_{i=1}^n y_i = (1/n)\sum_{i=1}^n \hat{y}_i$, i.e. the average of the fitted values is equal to the average of the responses. From the second normal equation, we can show that $\sum_{i=1}^n x_i\,e_i = 0$. This means that the predictor and the residuals are uncorrelated. Furthermore, from these properties we can show that $\sum_{i=1}^n \hat{y}_i\,e_i = 0$. This means that the residuals are also uncorrelated with the fitted values. This makes sense intuitively.

We found the line of best fit in the least squares sense. The next step in the regression analysis is to describe this fit. Since we minimized the sum of squared residuals as our criterion of best fit, we could use

$$\text{SSE} = \sum_{i=1}^n e_i^2 = \sum_{i=1}^n (y_i - \hat{y}_i)^2,$$

as a descriptive measure of fit. SSE is called the *error sum of squares.* It is generally difficult to judge what is a small error sum of squares (since it depends on the measurement scale).

We need to find a measure that is easier to interpret. To do so, we will perform an analysis of variance. The variability in the response is measured with the sample variance:

$$s_y^2 = \frac{1}{n-1} \sum_{i=1}^{n} (y_i - \overline{y})^2.$$

Example 15.1 (Part 2). Consider the number of colds data from Example 9.8. The number of colds varies from subject to subject. The sample variance is $s_y^2 = 7.882$. This measure of variability compares the responses to the mean response $\overline{y} = 9.75$.

If there is a linear association between x and y, then as the x-value moves away from its mean, the corresponding y-value tends to also move away from its mean. So we can use the line of best fit to explain some of the total variability in the responses. We decompose the total deviation into two components: an explained deviation and an unexplained deviation (also called the residual).

$$\begin{array}{ccccc} y_i - \overline{y} & = & (\widehat{y}_i - \overline{y}) & + & (y_i - \widehat{y}_i) \\ \text{total deviation} & = & \text{explained deviation} & + & \text{unexplained deviation} \end{array}$$

The sum of the squared total deviations is the *total sum of squares*:

$$\text{SST} = \sum_{i=1}^{n} (y_i - \overline{y})^2 = (n-1)\, s_y^2.$$

The total sum of squares is a measure of the total variability in the responses. The sum of the squared explained deviations is the *regression sum of squares*:

$$\text{SSR} = \sum_{i=1}^{n} (\hat{y}_i - \overline{y})^2 = \hat{\beta}^2\, (n-1)\, s_x^2.$$

To see this, note that:

$$\begin{aligned} \hat{y}_i - \overline{y} = \hat{\alpha} + \hat{\beta}\, x_i - \overline{y} &= \overline{y} - \hat{\beta}\, \overline{x} + \hat{\beta}\, x_i - \overline{y} \quad \text{by (15.2)} \\ &= \hat{\beta}(x_i - \overline{x}). \end{aligned}$$

The regression sum of squares is a measure of the variability that is explained by the regression. Using the fact that the residuals and the fitted values are uncorrelated and the residual average is equal to zero, one can show that the total sum of squares can be decomposed as follows:

$$\text{SST} = \text{SSR} + \text{SSE}.$$

The proportion of the total variability in the responses explained by the regression on the predictor is given by the *coefficient of determination*:

$$R^2 = \frac{\text{SSR}}{\text{SST}} = \frac{\hat{\beta}^2\,(n-1)\,s_x^2}{(n-1)\,s_y^2} = r_{xy}^2.$$

Note that the coefficient of determination is equal to the square of the sample correlation between x and y.

Example 15.1 (Part 3). For the number of colds data in Example 9.8, the sample correlation between the number of colds and the dosage is $r_{xy} = -0.63837$. Therefore, the proportion of the variability in the number colds explained by the regression on the dosage of vitamin C is $R^2 = 40.8\%$.

Example 15.2 (Part 1). Refer to the mother-daughter sample of size $n = 12$ from Example 9.7. The response variable y is the height of the daughter and the predictor variable x is the height of the mother. We summarize the data with the following sums: $\sum x_i = 1{,}951.0$, $\sum y_i = 1{,}923.0$, $\sum x_i^2 = 317{,}267.0$, $\sum x_i\,y_i = 312{,}702.0$ and $\sum y_i^2 = 308{,}403$. Using (15.2) and (15.3) to compute the least squares estimates, we get the following estimated line $\widehat{y} = 0.8107\,x + 28.4421$. Figure 15.2 gives the scatter plot of the pairs (x_i, y_i) and the estimated regression line.

The proportion of the total variability in the heights of daughters which is explained by the regression on the heights of the mothers is $R^2 = 18.2\%$.

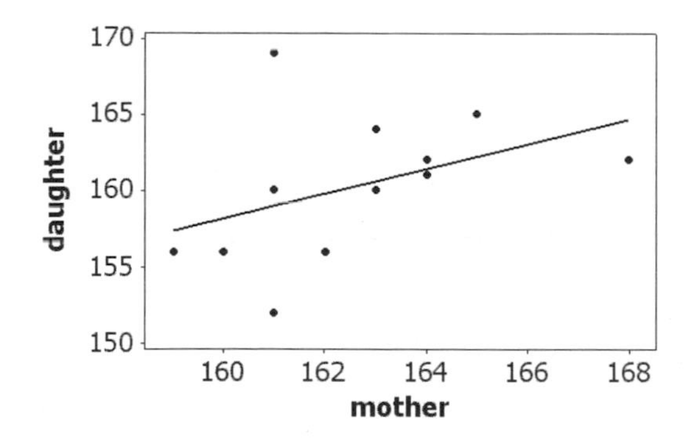

Fig. 15.2 Least squares line for the heights of mothers and daughters

15.2 Regression Model

In Section 15.1, we introduced the method of least squares to find a line of best fit which describes the linear association between a response variable y and a predictor x, based on a random sample of size n. Usually the analysis should not stop there. In this section we learn how to use the estimated line to predict future responses, or even perform hypotheses testing concerning the relationship between the response and the predictor variables.

We model the association between the response and the predictor as follows:

$$Y = \alpha + \beta\, x + \varepsilon, \tag{15.4}$$

where ε is a random variable called the *random error* such that $E(\varepsilon) = 0$ and $\mathrm{Var}(\varepsilon) = \sigma^2$. The model (15.4) is called a *simple linear regression model.* The term simple is used to emphasize the fact that there is only one predictor variable x.

To better understand the model, we investigate some properties of the simple linear regression model. Assume that the simple linear model (15.4) is valid. If we fix the predictor x, then the mean and the variance of the response are respectively:

$$\mu_{Y|x} = E(Y|x) = \alpha + \beta\, x \quad \text{and} \quad \mathrm{Var}(Y|x) = \sigma^2.$$

This means that there is a line such that for a fixed value x of the predictor, the responses are varying about the evaluation on this line. Furthermore the variance of the response Y at a fixed x is given by the error variance $\sigma^2 = \mathrm{Var}(\varepsilon)$, and this variance is the same for each x.

Example 15.1 (Part 4). Examine the scatter plot of the number of colds against the dosage of vitamin C in Section 15.1. The points do appear to be scattered about a line and the variability about this line seems to be similar for different x-values. Hence it appears to be reasonable to use the simple linear regression model (15.4) to relate the number of colds to the dosage of vitamin C. (We will encounter later in the sequel examples for which the simple linear model is not appropriate.)

Consider a random sample of size n of responses $Y_1, \ldots, Y_n$ that correspond to the predictor values $x_1, \ldots, x_n$. Using the method of least squares from Section 15.1, we obtain the least squares estimators for the regression coefficients β and α, respectively:

$$\widehat{\beta} = \sum_{i=1}^{n} \frac{(x_i - \overline{x})}{(n-1)s_x^2}\, Y_i \quad \text{and} \quad \widehat{\alpha} = \sum_{i=1}^{n} \left(\frac{1}{n} - \frac{(x_i - \overline{x})\, \overline{x}}{(n-1)\, s_x^2} \right) Y_i.$$

Since these estimators are linear combinations of the independent responses, we can compute their expectations and their variances. It turns out that $E(\widehat{\beta}) = \beta$, $E(\widehat{\alpha}) = \alpha$,

$$\operatorname{Var}(\widehat{\beta}) = \frac{\sigma^2}{(n-1)s_x^2} \quad \text{and} \quad \operatorname{Var}(\widehat{\alpha}) = \sigma^2 \left(\frac{1}{n} + \frac{\overline{x}^2}{(n-1)s_x^2} \right).$$

To estimate the mean response $\mu_{Y|x} = \alpha + \beta\, x$ at a given value x of the predictor, we use the least squares line $\hat{\mu}_{Y|x} = \widehat{\alpha} + \widehat{\beta}\, x$. It can be shown that $\overline{Y}$ and $\widehat{\beta}$ are uncorrelated. Using the properties of the least squares estimators, one can show that

$$E(\hat{\mu}_{Y|x}) = \alpha + \beta\, x = \mu_{Y|x} \quad \text{and} \quad \operatorname{Var}(\hat{\mu}_{Y|x}) = \sigma^2 \left(\frac{1}{n} + \frac{(x-\overline{x})^2}{(n-1)s_x^2} \right).$$

So, the least squares estimation leads to an unbiased estimation of the mean response for a given value x of the predictor. Notice that as x moves away from the average $\overline{x}$ of the predictor values in our sample, the estimate becomes less precise.

To describe the precision of least squares estimation we need to estimate the error variance σ^2. We can measure the variability about the least squares line with the *mean squared error* which is defined as

$$\text{MSE} = \frac{\text{SSE}}{n-2} = \frac{\sum_{i=1}^{n} (y_i - \hat{y}_i)^2}{n-2}.$$

Note that MSE is approximately the average squared deviation of the n responses, away from the least squares line. However instead of dividing by n, we divide by $n-2$ which corresponds to the number of degrees of freedom in this case. To estimate the variance about the line, we first have estimated the intercept and the slope of the line, which causes a loss of 2 degrees of freedom. It can be shown that MSE is an unbiased estimator of the error variance σ^2, that is

$$E(\text{MSE}) = \sigma^2.$$

As we collect the n paired observations $(x_1, y_1), \ldots, (x_n, y_n)$, a quick and easy way to compute the MSE is as follows:

$$\text{MSE} = \frac{\text{SST} - \text{SSR}}{n-2} = \frac{(n-1)\, s_y^2 - \hat{\beta}^2\, (n-1)\, s_x^2}{n-2}. \tag{15.5}$$

We are now ready to estimate the standard errors of the estimates:

$$s\{\widehat{\alpha}\} = \sqrt{\text{MSE} \left(\frac{1}{n} + \frac{\overline{x}^2}{(n-1)s_x^2} \right)}, \quad s\{\widehat{\beta}\} = \sqrt{\frac{\text{MSE}}{(n-1)s_x^2}},$$

and

$$s\{\hat{\mu}_{Y|x}\} = \sqrt{\text{MSE}\left(\frac{1}{n} + \frac{(x-\overline{x})^2}{(n-1)s_x^2}\right)}.$$

To use the regression analysis for confidence interval or hypothesis testing for the unknown regression parameters, we make an assumption of normality concerning the probability distribution of the response variable. More precisely, we assume that the responses $Y_1, \ldots, Y_n$ are independent random variables such that

$$Y_i = \alpha + \beta\, x_i + \varepsilon_i,$$

where ε_i follow a $N(0, \sigma^2)$ distribution. Assuming that the underlying assumptions of this model are valid, it can be shown that the following three random variables

$$\frac{\widehat{\alpha}-\alpha}{s\{\widehat{\alpha}\}}, \quad \frac{\widehat{\beta}-\beta}{s\{\widehat{\beta}\}} \quad \text{and} \quad \frac{\hat{\mu}_{Y|x}-\mu_{Y|x}}{s\{\hat{\mu}_{Y|x}\}} \tag{15.6}$$

have a $T(n-2)$ distribution. Using this fact, we can construct confidence intervals for the regression coefficients α and β, and also for a mean response $\mu_{Y|x}$ at a given value x of the predictor.

The arguments used to construct these intervals are the same as found in Section 10.2 to construct a confidence interval for a population mean. The confidence intervals for these parameters are all of the same form. A $(1-\alpha)\,100\%$ confidence interval is of the form:

$$\text{point estimate} \pm t\,(\text{estimated standard error}),$$

where t is a number found in Table 17.4 that satisfies $P(-t < T < t) = 1-\alpha$ and T has a $T(n-2)$ distribution.

Example 15.2 (Part 2). The response variable y is the daughter's height and the predictor variable x is the mother's height. The sample variances for the daughters' heights and for the mothers' heights are, respectively, $s_y^2 = 22.022727$ and $s_x^2 = 6.083333$. Using (15.5), we compute the estimate of the error variance: MSE $= 19.8269$.

Recall that the least-squares estimates of slope and intercept are $\widehat{\beta} = 0.8107$ and $\widehat{\alpha} = 28.4421$, respectively. The estimated standard errors for these estimates are, respectively,

$$s\{\widehat{\beta}\} = \sqrt{\frac{19.8269}{(12-1)(6.083333)}} = 0.5443$$

and

$$s\{\widehat{\alpha}\} = \sqrt{19.8269\left(\frac{1}{12} + \frac{(1,951/12)^2}{(12-1)(6.083333)}\right)} = 88.5079.$$

To build 95% confidence intervals for the slope β and the intercept α, we use $t = 2.228$. The 95% confidence intervals for β and α are, respectively,

$$\widehat{\beta} \pm t\, s\{\widehat{\beta}\} = [-0.40, 2.02] \quad \text{and} \quad \widehat{\alpha} \pm t\, s\{\widehat{\alpha}\} = [-168.75, 225.63].$$

A point estimate for the mean height of daughters whose mothers have a height of $x = 165$ cm is $\hat{\mu}_{Y|x=165} = \widehat{\alpha} + \widehat{\beta}\,(165) = 162.21$ cm. The corresponding estimated standard error is:

$$s\{\hat{\mu}_{Y|x=165}\} = \sqrt{19.8269\left(\frac{1}{12} + \frac{(165-(1951/12))^2}{(12-1)(6.083333)}\right)} = 1.8392.$$

A 95% confidence interval for the mean height of daughters whose mothers have a height of $x = 165$ cm is

$$\hat{\mu}_{Y|x=165} \pm t\, s\{\hat{\mu}_{Y|x=165}\} = [158.11, 166.31].$$

The three test statistics in (15.6) can also be used to test hypotheses concerning the parameters α, β or $\mu_{Y|x}$. These lead to t-tests with $n-2$ degrees of freedom. In particular, we commonly test the null hypothesis $H_0 : \beta = 0$ against $H_1 : \beta \neq 0$. This is called a *test for the significance of the regression.* Rejecting the null hypothesis leads to a conclusion of a significant linear effect of x. Failing to reject the null hypothesis could mean many things: (i) the test is not powerful enough to detect an important linear effect of x, and we need to increase the sample size; (ii) there is no linear relationship between the two variables, and so, x plays no role in explaining the variability in the response Y; or, (iii) the relationship between the two variables is not linear, and so, x could still be useful in explaining the variability in the response variable. To address the issue (i), we could construct a confidence interval for the slope and determine if the estimation is precise enough. To address issues (ii) and (iii), we produce a scatter plot of the pairs (x, y). In Example 15.3 below, we use a scatter plot to gain insight concerning the relationship between the response and the predictor variables.

Example 15.2 (Part 3). We test for the significance of the regression of the daughters' heights against the mothers' heights. We are testing $H_0 : \beta = 0$ against $H_1 : \beta \neq 0$. The observed value of the test statistic is

$$t_0 = \frac{\widehat{\beta} - 0}{s\{\widehat{\beta}\}} = \frac{0.8107 - 0}{0.5443} = 1.49.$$

Since this is a two-tailed test, the p-value is $P = 2\,P(T > 1.49)$, where T has $T(10)$ distribution. Referring to row $\nu = 10$ in Table 17.4, the value 1.49 falls between 1.372 and 1.812, which have areas to the right of 0.10 and 0.05. Thus, $0.10 < p\text{-value} < 0.20$. If the significance level of the test is $\alpha = 0.20$, then we reject H_0 and accept the alternative H_1 to conclude that there is a significant linear effect of the predictor x. However, if $\alpha = 0.10$, then we do not reject H_0 and conclude that the linear effect of x is not significant.

It is recommended that you always produce a scatter plot. The scatter plot is a useful *diagnostic tool.* It allows us to verify the underlying assumption of linearity between y and x as seen in the following example.

Example 15.3. To investigate the effect of a particular stimulant on reaction times, the researchers randomly assignment a dosage of the stimulant to the subjects. The treatment groups are 0 mg, 10 mg, 20 mg, 30 mg, 40 mg and 50 mg. Each group contains 10 subjects. The response y is the reaction time (in seconds) and the predictor x is the assigned dosage (in mg).

The least squares line is $\widehat{y} = 39.5311 - 0.07120\,x$, which is overlayed in the scatter plot given in Figure 15.3. Since the slope is negative, it appears that on average an increase in the dosage will decrease the reaction time.

The sample variances of the responses and predictors are $s_y^2 = 53.50067$ and $s_x^2 = 293.19209$. Only $R^2 = \text{SSR}/\text{SST} = \widehat{\beta}^2\,(n-1)s_x^2/[(n-1)s_y^2] = 2.8\%$ of the total variability in the reaction times is explained by the regression with the dosage of the stimulant. There appears to be little linear association between the two variables. We test for the significance of the regression.

The point estimate for the error variance σ^2 is

$$\text{MSE} = \frac{\text{SSE}}{n-2} = \frac{(n-1)s_y^2 - \widehat{\beta}^2\,(n-1)s_x^2}{n-2} = 52.9118.$$

To test $H_0 : \beta = 0$ against $H_1 : \beta \neq 0$, we evaluate the test statistic

$$t = \frac{\widehat{\beta} - 0}{s\{\widehat{\beta}\}} = \frac{\widehat{\beta}}{\sqrt{\text{MSE}/(n-1)s_x^2}} = -1.29.$$

The p-value is $2\,P(T > 1.29)$, where T has a $T(58)$ distribution. Since n is large, we use row $\nu = \infty$ in Table 17.4 to approximate the p-value. We obtain $0.1 < p\text{-value} < 0.2$. Using a statistical package, we find that $p\text{-value} = 0.203$. The p-value is large, so we should not reject the null hypothesis.

The investigators were prudent and were not ready to conclude that the stimulant has no effect on the reaction times. They produced the scatter plot of the pairs (x_i, y_i) (see Figure 15.3), and noticed that the relationship between y and x does not appear to be linear. Since one of the underlying assumptions of the simple linear model is that there is a linear association between the two variables, they concluded that simple linear regression is inappropriate in this case.

Using techniques which are beyond the scope of this textbook, the researchers fitted a quadratic response function. They obtain the following estimated quadratic response function $\widehat{y} = 48.7 - 1.44\,x + 0.0274x^2$, for which the corresponding coefficient of determination is $R^2 = 93\%$. This means that 93% of the variability in the reaction times is explained by the polynomial regression on the dosage of the stimulant.

It appears that there is a strong association between the reaction times and the dosage of the stimulant. It is just that this association is not linear.

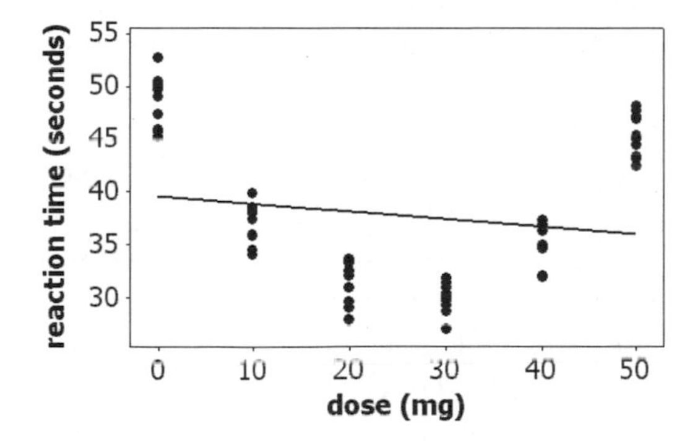

Fig. 15.3 The least squares line of reaction time

Another useful diagnostic tool is the *residual plot*, which is a plot of the residuals against the predictors or against the fitted values. It allows us to verify the underlying assumptions of linearity, and of homogeneity of the variance. Recall that we assumed, that regardless of the value x of the predictor, the variance of the response is equal to the constant σ^2. To verify the assumption of normal random errors, we can produce a normal probability plot of the residuals.

Example 15.4 (Part 1). Scientists want to construct a model for the fecundity (number of eggs per year) of a particular species of fish, as a function of its length x in centimeters.

From a sample of $n = 100$ observations, the scientists computed the coefficient of determination $R^2 = 79.8\%$. The p-value for the test for the significance of the regression was less than 0.0001. So a large proportion of the variability in the response was explained by the predictor, and the regression is highly significant. However as they investigated further, they determined that inferences with the simple linear model were inappropriate.

Figure 15.4 give the scatter plot of the fecundity against then length, with an overlay of the least squares line. To the right of the scatter plot, we find the residual plot of the residuals against the predictors.

The association between fecundity and length does not appear to be linear. This curvilinear tendency is more apparent in the residual plot. A systematic tendency in the residual plot is evidence against the underlying assumption of linearity of the simple linear regression model. Furthermore, the residuals appear to be more variable for larger fish. It appears that we have strong evidence that the error variance is not constant. The scientists decided that simple linear regression is not appropriate to analyze the relationship between fecundity and length.

Since fecundity appears to increase exponentially as a function of length, the scientists expressed fecundity on a logarithmic scale. The response variable y is log(fecundity) and the predictor x is length (in cm).

There appears to be a linear association between y and x, and the residuals also do not appear to vary much with x (see Figure 15.5). It is reasonable to use the simple linear regression model in this case. The least squares line is $\widehat{y} = 8.76 + 0.0741\,x$. The coefficient of determination is $R^2 = 88.6\%$ and the p-value of the test for the significance of the regression is less than 0.0001. The regression is highly significant.

We end the section with a discussion concerning prediction. We know how to estimate the mean response for a fixed value x of the predictor.

Example 15.2 (Part 4). We estimated that the height of daughters, whose mothers have a height of 165 cm, would be between 158.11 cm and

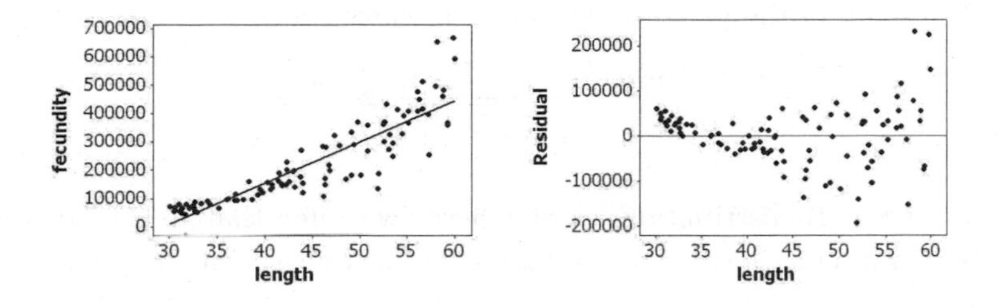

Fig. 15.4 Scatter and residual plot for fecundity against length

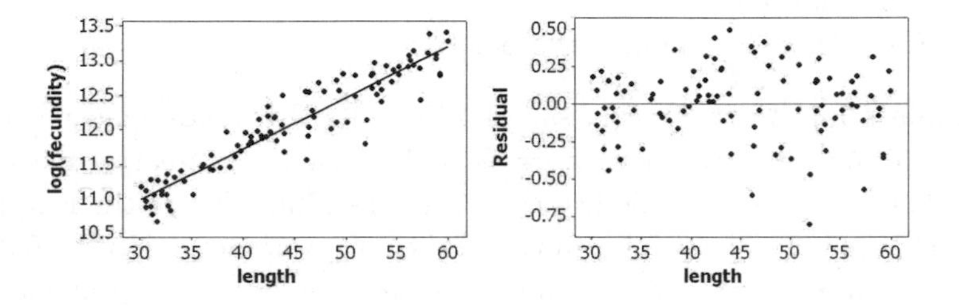

Fig. 15.5 Scatter and residual plot for log-fecundity against length

166.31, with a level of confidence of 95%.

Suppose that we want to predict the height of a randomly chosen daughter from this group, instead of estimating the mean of the group. To do so, we construct a prediction interval.

Let Y_{new} represent a new response for a fixed level x of the predictor. We can evaluate the corresponding value on the least squares line (constructed from a sample of n paired observations) as the predictor $\hat{Y}_{\text{new}} = \hat{\alpha} + \widehat{\beta}\, x$. The error of the prediction is $Y_{\text{new}} - \hat{Y}_{\text{new}}$. Assuming that the underlying conditions of the simple linear regression model hold, it can be shown that the expected value of the error of the prediction is $E(Y_{\text{new}} - \hat{Y}_{\text{new}}) = 0$ and that its variance is

$$\text{Var}(Y_{\text{new}} - \hat{Y}_{\text{new}}) = \sigma^2 + \sigma^2 \left(\frac{1}{n} + \frac{(x - \overline{x})^2}{(n-1)s_x^2} \right).$$

Standardizing the error of the prediction with the estimated error variance

MSE (instead of the variance σ^2), one can show that

$$\frac{Y_{\text{new}} - \hat{Y}_{\text{new}}}{s\{\text{pred}\}} = \frac{Y_{\text{new}} - \hat{Y}_{\text{new}}}{\sqrt{\text{MSE}\left(1 + \frac{1}{n} + \frac{(x-\overline{x})^2}{(n-1)s_x^2}\right)}}$$

has a $T(n-2)$ distribution. From here, we infer that a $(1-\alpha)\,100\%$ prediction interval for a new response at a fixed level x of the predictor is

$$\hat{y}_{\text{new}} \pm t\, s\{\text{pred}\} = \widehat{\alpha} + \widehat{\beta}\, x \pm t\sqrt{\text{MSE}\left(1 + \frac{1}{n} + \frac{(x-\overline{x})^2}{(n-1)s_x^2}\right)},$$

where t is a number such that $1 - \alpha = P(-t < T < t)$, and T follows a $T(n-2)$ distribution.

We end with two examples of prediction.

Example 15.4 (Part 2). The sample of $n = 100$ fish yields a mean length $\overline{x} = 44.67$ cm, and variance $s_x^2 = 84.143$. The least squares line $\widehat{y} = 8.76 + 0.0741\, x$ expresses the log-fecundity y as a function of the length x (in cm) of the fish. The point estimate of the error variance is MSE $= 0.060$.

Using Table 17.4, we get a number $t = 1.96$ that satisfies approximately $95\% = P(-t < T < t)$, where T follows a $T(n-2) = T(98)$ distribution. (Since n is large, we use row $\nu = \infty$ as an approximation.) A 95% prediction interval for the log-fecundity of a fish of $x = 50$ cm is

$$8.76 + 0.0741\,(50) \pm 1.96\sqrt{0.060\left(1 + \frac{1}{100} + \frac{(50 - 44.67)^2}{(100-1)(84.143)}\right)}$$
$$= [11.982, 12.948].$$

We exponentiate to obtain a 95% prediction interval for the fecundity of a fish of $x = 50$ cm:

$$[e^{11.982}, e^{12.948}] = [159,851; 419,996].$$

Example 15.1 (Part 5). The sample of $n = 20$ subjects has a mean dosage of $\overline{x} = 23.75$ and variance $s_x^2 = 360.20$. The least squares line $\widehat{y} = 12.0 - 0.0944\, x$ expresses the number y of colds in 3 years as a function of the daily dosage x (in mg) of vitamin C. The point estimate of the error variance is MSE $= 4.929$.

To verify the underlying assumptions of the simple linear regression model, we produce the normal probability plot of the residuals and the residual plot of the residuals against the dosage (see Figure 15.6).

There is no systematic pattern in the residuals, and the variability of the residuals per group appears to be similar. It appears that the underlying assumptions of linearity and constant error variance hold. In the normal probability plot, there are no pronounced systematic deviations from the normal line. So, it is reasonable to assume that the random errors are normally distributed. We can use the simple linear regression model for inferential purposes.

A 95% prediction interval for a subject given a daily dose of $x = 25$ mg is

$$12.0 - 0.0944\,(25) \pm 2.101\sqrt{4.929\left(1 + \frac{1}{100} + \frac{(25-23.75)^2}{(20-1)(360.20)}\right)}$$

$$= [4.86, 14.42],$$

where $t = 2.101$ is a number from row $\nu = n - 2 = 18$ in Table 17.4 such that $95\% = P(-t < T < t)$, and T has a $T(18)$ distribution.

Note that the sample range of the predictor variable is from 0 mg to 50 mg. We could predict a number of colds for a subject given a daily dosage of $x = 60$ mg or even $x = 75$ mg. However these values are outside the range of the values used to construct the model. Such predictions are called *extrapolations.*

We should be careful with extrapolations. We cannot be sure that the linear tendency continues to hold for values outside the scope of our model. Extrapolations at values far outside the scope of the model are unreliable.

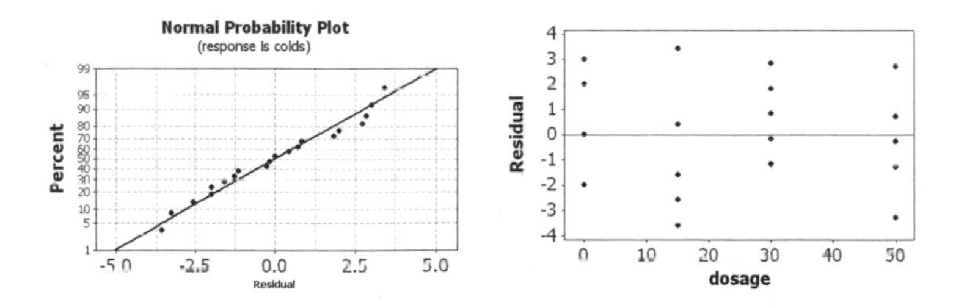

Fig. 15.6 Normal probability plot of the residuals and residual plot for number of colds against dosage of vitamin C

To summarize, in this section we introduced the simple linear regression model $Y = \alpha + \beta\, x + \varepsilon$, with the following underlying assumptions:

- statistical linear association between Y and x;

- the error variance $\sigma^2 = V(\varepsilon)$ is constant;
- the random errors are independent and normally distributed.

The scatter plot and the residual plot can be used as diagnostic tools to verify the assumption of linearity and variance homogeneity. To verify the assumption of normality, we can produce a normal probability plot of the residuals.

Once the underlying assumptions are verified, we can use the simple linear regression model for inference concerning the intercept α, the slope β, or the mean response $\mu_{Y|x}$ at a given fixed value x of the predictor. We can also use the model to predict a new response for a given fixed value of the predictor. We caution the user of regression to be aware of extrapolations.

15.3 Correlation

A correlation analysis is an assessment of the degree of linear association between two variables Y and X. It is closely related to the linear regression analysis, but the focus is on measuring the strength of the relationship instead of trying to describe the relationship functionally. In this section, we discuss inferences concerning a correlation coefficient. The readers should reacquaint themselves with the sample correlation

$$r_{xy} = \frac{s_{xy}}{s_x\, s_y} = \frac{[\sum_{i=1}^{n}(x_i - \overline{x})(y_i - \overline{y})]/(n-1)}{\sqrt{[\sum_{i=1}^{n}(x_i - \overline{x})^2/(n-1)][\sum_{i=1}^{n}(y_i - \overline{y})^2/(n-1)]}}$$

and its properties (see the end of Section 9.1).

The first step in a correlation analysis is to construct a scatter plot for assessing linearity. In Example 15.3, the sample correlation between the reaction time and the dosage of the stimulant is $r = \hat{\beta}\sqrt{s_x^2/s_y^2} = -0.1667$. This correlation is weak, but we can explain a very high proportion of the variation in the reaction times with a quadratic regression model of the dosage. So, in this case, the correlation is not a useful tool to measure the strength of the association between the two variables. However, if the association is linear, then the correlation does measure the degree of association between the variables.

Consider the heights of the mother-daughter pairs from Example 9.7 and the vitamin C experiment from Example 9.8. In these examples, the tendency between the two variables appears to be linear, hence a correlation is appropriate to measure the strength of association. For the above mentioned samples, the correlation between the heights of the mothers and the daughters is $r = 0.426$, and the correlation between the number of colds and the dosage of vitamin C is $r = -0.638$. These quantities were computed from their respective samples, and thus are point estimates of the population correlation between the involved variables.

Can we determine if the variables X and Y are correlated by taking the sampling error into account? We will see that under some underlying population assumptions, we can determine the significance of the correlation using simple linear regression.

Suppose that we have a random sample $(X_1, Y_1), \ldots, (X_n, Y_n)$ of size n, where $E(X) = \mu_X$, $E(Y) = \mu_Y$, $\text{Var}(X) = \sigma_X^2$, $\text{Var}(Y) = \sigma_X^2$, and the correlation between X and Y is

$$\rho = \frac{E[(X - \mu_X)(Y - \mu_Y)]}{\sigma_X \, \sigma_Y}.$$

Now suppose that there is a linear association between Y and X in the sense that $E(Y|X = x) = \alpha + \beta\, x$. Then, it can be shown that

$$\alpha = \mu_Y - \beta\, \mu_X \quad \text{and} \quad \beta = \rho\, \frac{\sigma_Y}{\sigma_X}.$$

Looking closely at the slope β, we notice that it is related to the correlation ρ. Actually, under the above assumption of linearity, the correlation is equal to zero if and only if the slope is zero. We can exploit this fact to develop a test for a non-zero correlation.

We want to test

$$\begin{cases} H_0 : \rho = 0 & [\text{ that is } X \text{ and } Y \text{ are uncorrelated}]; \\ H_1 : \rho \neq 0 & [\text{that is } X \text{ and } Y \text{ are correlated}]. \end{cases}$$

We use the following test statistic

$$R\, \frac{\sqrt{n-2}}{\sqrt{1 - R^2}} = \frac{\widehat{\beta}}{s\{\widehat{\beta}\}}, \tag{15.7}$$

where R is the sample correlation between X and Y, and $\widehat{\beta}$ is the slope of the least squares line when regressing Y against X. If we assume that $Y|X = x$ follows a normal distribution with mean $E(Y|x) = \alpha + \beta\, x$ and variance $\text{Var}(Y|x) = \sigma^2$, then under the null hypothesis that $\rho = 0$, we also have that $\beta = 0$. This is exactly the test for the significance of the regression. Under H_0, the sampling distribution $\widehat{\beta}/s\{\widehat{\beta}\}$ has a $T(n-2)$ distribution. It follows that the p-value of the test for a non-zero correlation between X and Y is

$$p\text{-value} = 2\, P(T > |t_0|),$$

where T has a $T(n-2)$ distribution, and t_0 is the observed value of the test statistic (15.7).

Once we measure the significance of the correlation, it is useful to construct a confidence interval for the true correlation ρ. We construct an approximate confidence interval based on *Fisher's z-transform*. It can be shown that for n large,

$$Z = \left\{\frac{1}{2}\ln\left[\frac{1+R}{1-R}\right] - \frac{1}{2}\ln\left[\frac{1+\rho}{1-\rho}\right]\right\} \Big/ \sqrt{\frac{1}{n-3}}$$

has approximately a $N(0,1)$ distribution. Hence a $(1-\alpha)\,100\%$ confidence interval for $\frac{1}{2}\ln[(1+\rho)(1-\rho)]$ is

$$\frac{1}{2}\ln\left(\frac{1+r}{1-r}\right) \pm \frac{z}{\sqrt{n-3}} = (a,b),$$

where z is a number such that $1-\alpha = P(-z < Z < z)$, and Z follows a $N(0,1)$ distribution. Applying an inverse transformation to the bounds of the confidence interval gives us a confidence interval for ρ. Therefore, a $(1-\alpha)\,100\%$ confidence interval for ρ is

$$\left(\frac{e^{2a}-1}{e^{2a}+1}, \frac{e^{2b}-1}{e^{2b}+1}\right).$$

Example 15.1 (Part 6). The correlation between the number of colds and the dosage of vitamin C is $r = -0.638$. To test $H_0 : \rho = 0$ against $H_1 : \rho \neq 0$, where ρ is the correlation coefficient between X and Y, we compute the observed value of the test statistic (15.7)

$$t_0 = -0.638\,\frac{\sqrt{20-2}}{\sqrt{1-(-0.638)^2}} = -3.515.$$

The p-value is $2\,P(T > |-3.515|) = 2\,P(T > 3.515)$, where T follows a $T(18)$ distribution. Since $P(T > 3.46) < 0.005$, then the p-value is less than 0.001. The p-value is very small so we can reject the null hypothesis and accept that correlation between the number of colds and the dosage of vitamin C is not zero.

To construct a 95% confidence interval for ρ, we start by constructing an approximate 95% confidence interval for $(1/2)\ln[(1+\rho)/(1-\rho)]$ which is

$$\begin{aligned}\frac{1}{2}\ln\left(\frac{1+r}{1-r}\right) \pm \frac{1.96}{\sqrt{n-3}} &= \frac{1}{2}\ln\left(\frac{1-0.638}{1+0.638}\right) \pm \frac{1.96}{\sqrt{20-3}}\\ &= (-1.23016, -0.27942).\end{aligned}$$

Thus, an approximate 95% confidence interval for the population correlation is ρ

$$\left(\frac{e^{2(-1.23016)}-1}{e^{2(-1.23016)}+1}, \frac{e^{2(-0.27942)}-1}{e^{2(-0.27942)}+1}\right) = (-0.843, -0.272).$$

In this example, we see the importance of interval estimation. The point estimate for the correlation is $r = -0.638$, which hints at a moderately strong correlation. However, taking the sampling error into account, we cannot conclude that the correlation is strong since it can be as small as -0.27. To obtain a more precise estimate, we must collect a larger sample. The next example also illustrates the need for interval estimates.

Example 15.2 (Part 5). The correlation between the mothers' heights and the daughters' heights is $r = 0.426$. There appears to be a moderate association between the two variables. However in Example 15.2 (Part 3), we tested for the significance of the regression of the daughters' heights against the mothers' heights. The p-value was larger than 0.10. Since this test is equivalent to the test for a non-zero correlation, we cannot reject the null hypothesis of a zero correlation.

The sampling error must be large. To investigate, we construct a 95% confidence interval for the population correlation ρ. A 95% confidence interval for $(1/2)\ln[(1+\rho)/(1-\rho)]$ is:

$$\begin{aligned}\frac{1}{2}\ln\left(\frac{1+r}{1-r}\right) \pm \frac{1.96}{\sqrt{n-3}} &= \frac{1}{2}\ln\left(\frac{1+0.426}{1-0.426}\right) \pm \frac{1.96}{\sqrt{12-3}} \\ &= (-0.198334, 1.108333).\end{aligned}$$

Thus an approximate 95% confidence interval for the population correlation ρ is:

$$\left(\frac{e^{2(-0.198334)}-1}{e^{2(-0.198334)}+1}, \frac{e^{2(1.108333)}-1}{e^{2(1.108333)}+1}\right) = (-0.196, 0.803)$$

We conclude that the estimate of the correlation between the mothers' heights and the daughters' heights is not precise. To obtain a better estimate, we need a larger sample.

As we developed the test for a non-zero correlation, we used the conditional distribution of Y given $X = x$, and we assumed that the simple linear regression model was appropriate. Thus, the residual analysis discussed in Section 15.2 can be used to verify the underlying assumptions of the correlation analysis. In Example 15.1 (Part 7) below, we discuss the verification of the underlying assumptions for the correlation analysis from Example 15.1 (Part 6).

Note that the correlation is the same regardless of which variable plays the role of the response or of the predictor. Furthermore, if the underlying assumptions of the simple regression model of Y regressed on X are not satisfied, we can try to regress X on Y. If the underlying assumptions for the latter model are satisfied, then we have verified the assumptions for the test of a non-zero correlation.

Example 15.1 (Part 7). We discuss the verification of the underlying assumptions for the correlation analysis from Example 15.1 (Part 6). Refer to Example 15.1 (Part 5) for the normal probability plot of the residuals and the residual plot against the predictor x. The normal probability plot appears to have a linear tendency, so it is reasonable to assume that the random error is normal. From the residual plot, the errors seem to be dispersed for different x-values. Thus, it is reasonable to assume that the error variance is constant.

We end this section with a short discussion on *causation*. Scientists generally want to establish causality relationship, i.e. a relationship in which the response (or effect) is a consequence of a cause (or causal factor). The scientific method can be used to establish a cause-and-effect relationship. The method involves performing experiments in which we can control the cause and the possible causal factors, and observe a significant effect. However, in biology and medicine, it is often unethical to assign a factor to a unit. For example, it is unethical to ask someone to smoke two cigarettes a day. Nevertheless, there are acceptable methods that can be used to distinguish causal from noncausal associations. Refer to Chapter 2 in [49] for a discussion on establishing causality in the context of epidemiology.

An aspect that is important for a causal association is the strength of association. If there is a causal relationship, then there is an association between the cause and effect. Therefore, a strong correlation between two variables can hint at the existence of a causal relationship. But a large correlation alone is not proof of causation.

Let us consider an example. Say we select a few communities at random, and we measure the correlation between the number of bananas consumed in a week per capita and the prevalence of a disease. Say the confidence interval for the correlation is $[-0.9; -0.85]$. We have observed a strong correlation between the two variables. Does this mean that eating more bananas causes the risk of developing the disease to decrease? It is doubtful. In this case, it is likely that there are lurking variables (such as a healthy lifestyle) that are causes of both eating more bananas and the decreased risk of disease.

A significant correlation between two variables is not sufficient evidence for a cause-and-effect relationship, however it does hint at the possibility of the existence of such a relationship. A significant correlation between two variables is evidence of an association between the two variables.

15.4 Problems

Problem 15.1. The height of a child as an adult can be predicted using the child's height at the age of 2. The following table gives the heights of 20 women (in cm), as adults and at the age of 2:

adult height (y)	height at age of 2 (x)	adult height (y)	height at age of 2 (x)
164.6	86.4	158.3	83.1
166.1	87.6	159.8	84.5
167.4	88.9	160.6	85.2
163.8	85.7	162.5	84.3
162.9	84.1	173.5	93.9
168.1	89.0	171.9	92.7
169.3	90.1	165.3	85.2
167.4	87.2	164.1	84.2
168.5	88.3	167.5	86.3
165.9	86.3	175.3	95.2

For this data, we have:

$$\sum_{i=1}^{20} y_i = 3,322.8, \quad \sum_{i=1}^{20} x_i = 1748.2 \quad \sum y_i^2 = 552,414.5$$

$$\sum_{i=1}^{20} x_i^2 = 153,028, \quad \sum_{i=1}^{20} x_i y_i = 290,710.1$$

(a) Calculate the estimated least squares line.

(b) Find the sample correlation between the height as an adult and the height at the age of 2. What is the proportion of the total variability in the adult heights explained by the regression on the height at age 2?

(c) Estimate the mean height of a girl as an adult, whose height at age 2 is 87.2 cm.
(d) Give a 95% confidence interval for the mean height of a girl as an adult, whose height at age 2 is 84 cm.

Problem 15.2. Systolic arterial blood pressure (SBP) and diastolic arterial blood pressure (DBP) frequently display a linear relationship characterized by the systolic-versus-diastolic slope and the sample correlation (see [25]). The following table gives the SBP and the DBP for 15 men aged between 40 and 65:

SBP (y)	DBP (x)	SBP (y)	DBP (x)
112	63	156	100
120	69	124	82
135	70	99	56
142	82	105	65
132	76	124	73
115	67	144	89
119	71	134	76
128	73		

(a) Calculate the mean SBP and the mean DBP for this sample.
(b) Calculate the sample covariance s_{xy}, the sample variances s_x^2, s_y^2, and the sample correlation r_{xy}.
(c) Give the line of the best fit which expresses the SBP as a function of the DBP.
(d) Give the 95% confidence intervals for the slope β and the intercept α of the line of the best fit from (c).
(e) Give the point estimate and the 90% confidence interval for the SBP of a man of age between 40 and 65, whose DBP is equal to 75.

Problem 15.3. Since Confederation, the Canadian population has been growing steadily. The following table gives the population of Canada (in millions) since 1951. The data is taken from Statistics Canada website. We denote by y the Canadian population and x the year. We have:

$$\sum_{i=1}^{30} x_i = 59,400, \quad \sum_{i=1}^{30} y_i = 730.381, \quad \sum_{i=1}^{30} x_i y_i = 1,449,110$$

$$\sum_{i=1}^{n} x_i^2 = 117,620,990, \quad \sum_{i=1}^{30} y_i^2 = 18,756.71$$

Year	Population	Year	Population	Year	Population
1951	14.009	1961	18.239	1971	21.963
1953	14.845	1963	18.931	1973	22.494
1955	15.698	1965	19.644	1975	23.143
1957	16.610	1967	20.500	1977	23.727
1959	17.483	1969	21.001	1979	24.203

Year	Population	Year	Population	Year	Population
1981	24.821	1991	27.945	2001	31.012
1983	25.367	1993	28.682	2003	31.676
1985	25.843	1995	29.303	2005	32.359
1987	26.449	1997	29.965	2007	33.115
1989	27.056	1999	30.404	2009	33.894

(a) Construct a scatterplot of the data. Give the estimated regression line of the population as a function of the year.
(b) Calculate the sample correlation r_{xy}. Interpret the result.
(c) What proportion of the total variability in the responses can be explained by regression?
(d) Calculate the sums of squares SST, SSR and SSE.
(e) Give a point estimate for the error standard deviation σ.

Problem 15.4. A large study was conducted to test the hypothesis that the skeletal muscle mass of women reduces with age. All women involved in the study had a body mass index of at most 35. For each of the 125 women participating in this study, the researchers recorded their total skeletal muscle mass (in kg) and their age (in years). The data are found in the file SkeletalMass.txt. The first column gives the skeletal muscle mass and the second column gives the age.
(a) Construct a scatterplot of the data. Give the estimated regression line of the skeletal muscle mass as a function of age.
(b) Calculate the sample correlation r_{xy}. Interpret the result.
(c) What proportion of the total variability in the responses can be explained by regression?
(d) Give a point estimate for the error standard deviation σ.
(e) Perform a residual analysis. Do the underlying assumptions of the simple linear regression model appear to hold?
(f) Test $H_0 : \rho = 0$ against $H_1 : \rho \neq 0$, where ρ is the population correlation between the skeletal muscle mass and age. Use a level of $\alpha = 0.05$.
(g) Compute a 95% confidence interval for ρ.

Problem 15.5. Bears play a role in the transfer of marine isotopes, in particular those taken from salmon, into the terrestrial ecosystem (see [30]). The values of the nitrogen isotope signature $\delta^{15}N$ (in per mil) measured from a certain foliage are modeled as a function of the distance from the river (in metres). Below are the data from a river with few bears and little to no salmon.

distance	50	100	150	200	250	300	350	400
$\delta^{15}N$	−3.48	−4.02	−3.00	−3.24	−3.96	−3.80	−3.14	−3.80

(a) Produce a scatter plot and compute the least squares line describing the value of the nitrogen isotope signature as a function of the distance from the river.
(b) Calculate the sums of squares SST, SSR and SSE.
(c) Give a point estimate for the error standard deviation σ.
(d) What proportion of the total variability in the responses can be explained by regression?
(e) Calculate the sample correlation r_{xy} and compute a 95% confidence interval for the population correlation ρ between the value of the nitrogen isotope signature and the distance from the river. Can we conclude that the value of the nitrogen isotope signature and the distance from the river are correlated?

Problem 15.6. Continue with the situation in Problem 15.5. Consider now the following data from a river with few bears and an abundant salmon population.

distance	50	75	100	125	150	200	225
$\delta^{15}N$	0.18	−0.97	−1.74	−1.96	−2.13	−2.31	−2.65
distance	250	300	325	350	375	400	
$\delta^{15}N$	−2.53	−2.52	−2.55	−2.59	−2.71	−2.87	

(a) Produce a scatter plot and compute the least squares line describing the value of the nitrogen isotope signature as a function of the distance from the river.
(b) Use the residuals from part (a) to produce a normal probability plot of the residuals and a residual plot. Use these plots to perform diagnostics of the underlying assumptions of the simple linear model. What are your findings?
(c) Because there is an abundant salmon population, but few bears for the nitrogen transfer, it is hypothesized that the value of the nitrogen isotope

signature is correlated with the inverse distance from the river. We transform the data by defining the predictor $x = 1/\text{distance}$. Produce a scatter plot and compute the least squares line describing the values of the nitrogen isotope signature as a function of x. What are your findings?
(d) What proportion of the total variability in the values of the nitrogen isotope signature can be explained by regression on $x = 1/\text{distance}$?
(e) Use the residuals from part (c) to produce a normal probability plot of the residuals and a residual plot. Use these plots to perform diagnostics of the underlying assumptions of the simple linear model. What are your findings?
(f) Can we conclude that the value of the nitrogen isotope signature is correlated with the inverse distance from the river? Use the level $\alpha = 0.05$.
(g) Compute a 95% confidence interval for the population correlation ρ between the value of the nitrogen isotope signature and the inverse distance from the river.

Problem 15.7. With an increase in human activity in bear habitats, there are more human-bear interactions (see [1]). The following data were collected over a few years in the back country of a particular park. They represent the number of human-bear interactions and the number of people using a shuttle bus during a two-week period.

Number of Bus Users	Human-Bear Interactions	Number of Bus Users	Human-Bear Interactions
1,750	1	14,000	16
2,000	1	14,025	10
5,880	2	14,035	8
6,000	2	14,250	12
7,775	2	15,004	10
10,002	4	15,250	12
10,025	5	15,300	9
10,035	3	15,750	11
11,050	5	15,750	20
12,004	9	16,000	12

(a) Produce a scatter plot and compute the least squares line describing the number of human-bear interactions as a function of the number of bus users. Does the association appear to be linear?
(b) Use the residuals from part (a) to produce a normal probability plot of the residuals and a residual plot. Use these plots to perform diagnostics

of the underlying assumptions of the simple linear model. What are your findings?
(c) Apply a logarithm transformation to the response by defining a new response variable $y = ln$(number of interactions). Produce a scatter plot and compute the least squares line describing y as a function of the number of bus users. Does the association appear to be linear?
(d) Use the residuals from part (c) to produce a normal probability plot of the residuals and a residual plot. Use these plots to perform diagnostics of the underlying assumptions of the simple linear model. What are your findings?
(e) Using the least squares line from part (c), predict the number of human-bear interactions for a two-week period in which there are 8,000 shuttle bus users. Construct the corresponding 95% prediction interval and interpret the result.
(f) Using the least squares line from part (c), estimate the mean number of human-bear interactions for a two-week period in which there are 8,000 shuttle bus users. Construct the corresponding 95% confidence interval and interpret the result.

Did you know that? *More than two thirds of world's plant species are found in the tropical rainforests, which are renowned for their massive bio-diversity. Rainforests, once covered 14% of the earth's land surface, now cover only 6%. Nearly half of the world's species of plants, animals and microorganisms will be destroyed or severely threatened over the next 25 years, due to rainforest deforestation. Experts estimate that the last remaining rainforests could be consumed in less than 40 years. The Tropical Plants Database is an international project dedicated to providing accurate and factual information on the plants of the Amazon Rainforest, created by the joint efforts of botanists, ethnobotanists, health professionals and phytochemists. More information about this project can be found at http://www.rain-tree.com/plants.htm.*

Chapter 16

Supplementary Problems (Statistics)

Problem 16.1. The following data gives the IQ scores for 8 adults

$$105 \quad 87 \quad 102 \quad 75 \quad 125 \quad 116 \quad 114 \quad 94.$$

Find the normal scores for this data. Is it reasonable to assume that the data comes from a normal distribution?

Problem 16.2. All Canadian ice shelves are attached to Ellesmere Island, in the Nunavut territory. The first observations about the extent of the Ellesmere ice shelf were recorded in 1906, during an expedition lead by Robert Peary. It is estimated that the shelves reduced by ninety percent in the 20th century. In the past 50 years, the area became the subject of intensive research on climate change (see [59]). The data below gives the annual total amount of precipitation in mm (water equivalent) recorded for Alert Station during the period 1967-1997:

Year	Precipitation	Year	Precipitation	Year	Precipitation
1967	170	1978	140	1989	177
1968	295	1979	103	1990	168
1969	200	1980	176	1991	175
1970	165	1981	125	1992	186
1971	140	1982	126	1993	140
1972	190	1983	204	1994	147
1973	195	1984	196	1995	174
1974	142	1985	98	1996	155
1975	138	1986	123	1997	195
1976	148	1987	124		
1977	110	1988	152		

(a) Calculate the mean and the standard deviation for this data set.
(b) Find the median and quartiles for this data set. Construct the boxplot and identify the outliers, if they exist.
(c) Can we assume that the annual amount of precipitation is normally distributed? Justify your answer.

Problem 16.3. Mount St. Helens is an active volcano situated in the Pacific Northwest region of the United States, which had a powerful eruption on May 18, 1980. The region around the volcano became a national park in 1982. Since the eruption, the size of the fish in Spirit Lake at the bottom of the volcano seems to have increased. In 2010, a sample of 30 rainbow trouts had an average weight of 2.3 lb and a sample standard deviation of 4 lb. Is there enough evidence that 30 years after the eruption, the average weight of the trouts is higher than the pre-eruption average weight of 1.9 lb? (Assume that the fish weight has a normal distribution.)

Problem 16.4. A WBC count is a blood test which measures the number of white blood cells. Normal values for adults are between 4 and 9 thousands per cubic millimeter (K/mm^3). Certain corticosteroid drugs may increase the value of the WBC count. The following data gives the WBC count for 10 persons who used a corticosteroid drug for 7 days:

6.5 7.8 9.5 10.1 11.3 6.7 5.5 8.7 6.4 12.1

Using this data, is there enough evidence that the drug increases the white blood cell count above the level of 9? Justify your answer using a test of hypothesis at level $\alpha = 0.05$.

Problem 16.5. The purpose of the study [17] was to investigate whether exposure to light at night may increase the risk of breast cancer, by suppressing the normal nocturnal production of melatonin by the pineal gland, which in turn could increase the release of estrogen by the ovaries. The case patients were 813 women aged 20 to 74 years with a new diagnostic of breast cancer. The control subjects were 792 women aged 20 to 74 years with no history of breast cancer. The subject was considered to experience a pattern of "nonpeak sleep" if she reported the following (at least once a week): 1) turning off the lights to go to sleep after 2:00 a.m., 2) rising for the day before 1:00 a.m., or 3) not going to bed at all. 104 of the case patients and 91 of the control subjects reported having experienced a pattern of "nonpeak sleep" in the 10 years before the study. Can we argue that the proportion of women with a pattern of "nonpeak sleep" is higher in the breast cancer population? To justify your answer, use an appropriate test of hypothesis at level $\alpha = 0.10$.

Problem 16.6. The study [10] examined the influence of spraying with an insecticide called carbaryl on the nesting, laying and hatching of birds in nesting boxes, for four species of birds. Records from 5 years prior to spraying (1960-1964) were compared with the observations made after the spraying which took place in the nesting season of 1965. For the tree swallow, among the 124 eggs laid in the 5 years before the spray, 108 were fertile and 104 resulted in surviving young birds. In the summer of 1965, among the 22 laid eggs by the tree swallows, 19 were fertile and 16 resulted in surviving young birds.
(a) Can we say that the fertility rate of the tree swallows dropped significantly due to the spraying? Justify your answer using a 95% confidence interval and a test of hypothesis at level $\alpha = 0.05$.
(b) Is there enough evidence that the survival rate of the young tree swallows dropped after the spraying? Justify your answer using a 95% confidence interval and a test of hypothesis at level $\alpha = 0.05$. (The survival rate refers to the proportion of eggs which result in surviving birds, among the fertile eggs.)

Problem 16.7. Most commercial shampoos contain a potent de-greaser called Sodium Lauryl Sulphate (SLS), which could be acting as an irritant to the scalp, when penetrating into the hair follicles left open by the normal cycle of hair loss. In the study [62], the skin's response to SLS was measured on a sample of 9 male volunteers. Each individual received a total of four 8 mm Finn Chambers, two on the mid-volar area of each forearm. One chamber of each arm was filled with the irritant (15 μl SLS), while the other contain a similar quantity of water vehicle control. The patch tests were left in contact with the skin for 48 hours. The intensity of the irritant reactions was visually assessed for erythema on a scale of 0 to 4, with 0 for no visible reaction, and 4 for intense erythema. SLS induced inflammation in most individuals, with a mean score of 3.0. The water vehicle control produced a slight reaction in some individuals with a mean score of 0.5. Assuming that the standard deviation of the differences between the SLS score and the control score was $s_d = 1.5$, can we conclude that SLS acts as an irritant to the skin? Justify your answer using a 95% confidence interval and a test of hypothesis at level $\alpha = 0.05$.

Problem 16.8. In viticulture, the yield is the amount of wine that is produced per unit surface of vineyard. The yield can be improved using fertilizers. The following data gives the yield for 10 randomly selected acres in a vineyard in two subsequent years, using the traditional fertilizer in the first year, and an organic fertilizer in the second year. The yield is expressed in tons of wine per acre.

	Traditional Fertilizer	Organic Fertilizer
Acre 1	3.42	3.31
Acre 2	3.50	3.35
Acre 3	3.47	3.43
Acre 4	3.24	3.31
Acre 5	3.56	3.40
Acre 6	3.57	3.49
Acre 7	3.25	3.28
Acre 8	3.33	3.28
Acre 9	3.52	3.46
Acre 10	3.46	3.42

Compare the average yield per acre for the two fertilizers, using a test of hypothesis at level $\alpha = 0.01$. Is there enough evidence that the traditional fertilizer produces a larger yield?

Problem 16.9. Artificial night lighting affects the natural behavior of many species of animals. The purpose of the study [47] was to see if artificial light at night may interfere with the ability of migratory birds to orient themselves. Turning off the lights is not a feasible solution for most offshore installations due to safety regulations. The area used for this study was the uninhabited Eastern cape of the barrier island Ameland (Dutch Wadden Sea). The following table gives the numbers of groups of birds which were attracted to the light source, depending on the light color (with peak wavelength in nm) and the sky conditions.

	Night conditions		
Light source	Clear sky	Overcast conditions	Total
white (diffuse)	38	156	194
red (670 nm)	13	24	37
green (535 nm)	8	77	85
blue (455 nm)	37	38	75
Total	96	295	391

The table suggests that birds are significantly disturbed by the white light in the overcast conditions, and not disturbed by the green light under the clear sky. Can we say that the proportions of birds affected by one type of light are the same under the clear sky and the overcast conditions? (Hint: Use a test of homogeneity at level $\alpha = 0.05$, even if the column totals are not fixed by the researchers.)

Problem 16.10. Optometrists recommend that school-age children should not watch television more that 1 hour per day. The following table gives the scores on a basic vision test for two groups of children: the first group consists of children who watch television more than 1 hour per day, the second group consists of children who watch television less that 1 hour per day.

	Score on the vision test		
Hours of TV time/day	poor	normal	Total
more than 1 hour	23	102	125 (fixed)
less than 1 hour	17	108	125 (fixed)
Total	40	210	250

(a) Give estimates for the proportions of children with poor vision score in the two groups. Give a 95% confidence interval for the difference between these two proportions. Interpret the result.
(b) Is there enough evidence that the proportion of children with normal vision score is higher in the second group? Use a test of hypothesis at level $\alpha = 0.05$.
(c) Using a test of homogeneity, verify if the proportions of children with poor vision scores are the same in the two groups. Use the level $\alpha = 0.05$.

Problem 16.11. The Healthy Eating Index (HEI) is a score on a scale of 1 to 100 which measures the intake of ten dietary components. A diet with a score greater than 80 is considered "good", whereas a diet with a score of less than 50 is considered "poor". It was found that children's school performance is directly related to the amount of nutrients in their diet, and even a moderate lack of nutrients can have lasting effects on their school performance. The following table gives the HEI score together with the score on a school performance test for a sample of 15 children in grade 6.

School Test (y)	HEI (x)	School Test (y)	HEI (x)
64	55	58	46
87	90	77	62
32	40	35	30
69	85	99	92
13	21	85	93
19	15	24	45
90	95	83	80
46	53		

(a) Give the estimated regression line $y = \hat{\alpha} + \hat{\beta}x$.
(b) Find the estimated standard errors for $\hat{\beta}$ and $\hat{\alpha}$.
(c) Find the 95% confidence intervals for the slope and the intercept of the regression line.
(d) Perform a test for the significance of the regression at level $\alpha = 0.01$.

Problem 16.12. The Giant Panda is an endangered species, due to the loss of its natural bamboo forest habitat, and a very low birthrate. In 2007, there were 266 Giant Pandas living in captivity, and an estimated 1,600 living in the wild. The primary method of breeding in captivity is by artificial insemination. A Giant Panda cub is extremely small, and because of this, it is difficult for the mother to protect it. The following data gives the gestation period x (in days) and the cub weight y (in g) at birth for a sample of 18 Giant Panda cubs born in captivity:

Weight (y)	Gestation period (x)	Weight (y)	Gestation period (x)
125	160	130	155
95	93	103	132
116	145	118	158
105	126	97	103
129	160	124	153
109	145	115	110
119	116	95	98
102	98	124	130
123	151	120	149

For these data, we have: $\bar{x} = 132.33, \bar{y} = 113.83, s_x^2 = 567.882, s_y^2 = 138.029, s_{xy} = 227.353$.
(a) Find the line of best fit in the least squares sense.
(b) Calculate the sample correlation r_{xy} and the coefficient of determina-

tion R^2. Interpret the value of R^2.
(c) Give an estimate for the error variance σ^2.
(d) Give a point estimate and a 99% confidence interval for the mean weight of a cub at birth, whose gestation period was 113 days.

Problem 16.13. Paracetamol (acetaminophen) is the most commonly used analgesic in young children. Some evidence suggests that ingestion of paracetamol in early life may cause asthma in some children. In the study [44], 495 children with a family history of allergic disease have been exposed to paracetamol in the first two years of life. It was found that 148 of these children have developed asthma between the age of 6 and 7.
(a) Give a 95% confidence interval for the proportion p of children with asthma, in the general population of children who were exposed to paracetamol in early life and have a family history of allergic disease.
(b) It is estimated that among the children with a family history of allergic disease, 25% have asthma. Is there enough evidence that the proportion p is higher than 25%? Use a test of hypothesis at level $\alpha = 0.01$.

Problem 16.14. To estimate the density of caribou in a particular region, the area is divided into 260 cells of equal size. Using areal surveillance, the number of caribou per cell is estimated. The data are given in the file caribou.txt.
(a) Construct the histogram for the number of caribou per cell. Describe the shape of the distribution.
(b) Would you recommend using the median or the mean to describe the center of the distribution?
(c) Describe the center of the distribution.
(d) Construct the box plot for the number of caribou per cell. Are there any outliers?
(e) Apply a log transformation to the number of caribou per cell. Construct a histogram for the transformed data. Describe the shape of the distribution. Are the mean and the standard deviation of the transformed values meaningful measurements of the center and the spread of the distribution of the log-number of caribou per cell?
(f) Using the mean and the standard deviation of the log-number of caribou per cell, compute the geometric mean and the geometric standard deviation of the number of caribou per cell.
(g) Summarize the geometric mean and the geometric standard deviation of the number of caribou per cell with an interval.

Problem 16.15. Consider two independent populations with means μ_1 and μ_2, respectively. The population variances are denoted by σ_1^2 and σ_2^2, respectively. Let $\overline{X}_i$ denote the sample mean for a sample of size n_i from the ith population, for $i = 1, 2$. Use the results from Section 9.2, to answer the following questions.
(a) Show that $\overline{X}_1 - \overline{X}_2$ is an unbiased estimator of $\mu_1 - \mu_2$.
(b) Show that $\text{Var}(\overline{X}_1 - \overline{X}_2) = \sigma_1^2/n_1 + \sigma_2^2/n_2$.
(c) If both populations are normal with $\mu_1 = 10$, $\mu_2 = 8$ and $\sigma_1^2 = \sigma_2^2 = 5$, and the sample sizes are $n_1 = n_2 = 10$, give the distribution of $\overline{X}_1 - \overline{X}_2$ and compute $P(\overline{X}_1 - \overline{X}_2 > 1.5)$.

Problem 16.16. A large study involved 524 households. For each household, the concentration of arsenic in the water (in $\mu g/l$) was measured. The data are given in the file ArsenicConcentrations.txt. The table below gives the mean and standard deviation for the arsenic concentration measurements and their natural logarithm.

Variable	Total Count	Mean	StDev
concentration	524	0.8441	2.1014
log-concentration	524	−1.3193	1.5200

Figure 16.1 gives the histogram of the concentrations of arsenic (on the left), and the histogram of the log-concentrations of arsenic (on the right).
(a) Give point estimates for the mean and the geometric mean of the concentration of arsenic. (Hint: The geometric mean of a measurement X is defined as the exponential of the mean of $\ln X$, i.e. $G = e^{E(\ln X)}$.)
(b) Construct a 95% confidence interval for the mean concentration of arsenic.
(c) Compute a 95% confidence interval for the mean log-concentration of arsenic. By exponentiating the limits of this interval, obtain a 95% confidence interval for the geometric mean of the concentration of arsenic.
(d) Comparing the confidence intervals from (b) and (c), which one do you think it describes better the center of the distribution of concentrations of arsenic? Why?

Problem 16.17. The authors of [60] found that the inefficient transport of iron from the root to the above-ground portion of a tomato mutant is controlled by a single recessive genetic factor. By crossing iron-inefficient mutants (ff) with normal plants (FF), they obtained a first generation F_1 of tomatoes in which all plants were normal (as expected). The plants

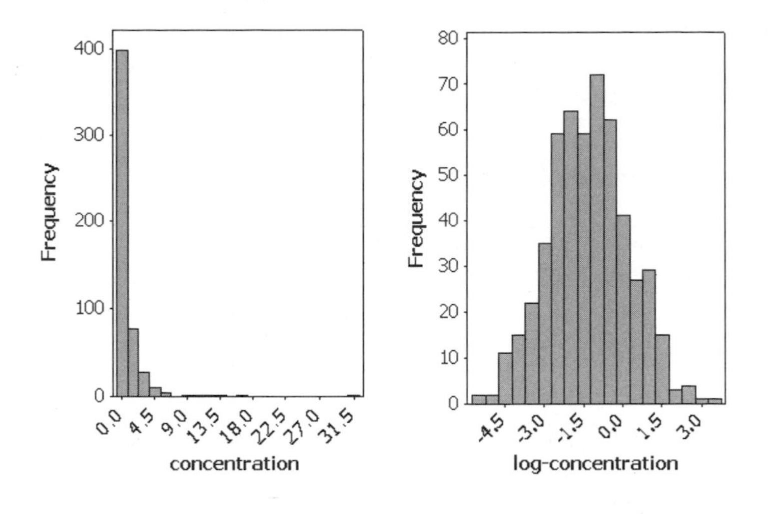

Fig. 16.1 Histograms: Concentration and log-concentration of arsenic

in the F_1 generation were crossed with one another, to produce a second generation F_2. The F_2 generation consisted of 245 tomatoes, among which 58 were iron-inefficient. Using these data, is there enough evidence to reject the single factor hypothesis? Use the level $\alpha = 0.05$. (Hint: Setup the hypotheses in terms of the probability p that a plant in the F_2 generation is iron-inefficient, assuming that the phenotype is controlled by a single recessive genetic factor.)

Problem 16.18. A public official believes that the mean household water use is 1,315 liters per day. A study of water usage involved a random sample of twenty five households. The data are given below. Assume that the household water use is normally distributed.

1316	1341	1303	1322	1335
1306	1320	1307	1352	1344
1329	1342	1301	1317	1311
1328	1290	1322	1310	1348
1324	1322	1339	1334	1369

(a) Using these data, is there enough evidence to conclude that the mean household water use is not 1,315 liters per day? Use $\alpha = 0.05$.
(b) Construct a 90% confidence interval for the mean household water use per day.

Problem 16.19. Methods for determining the fat content of foods are discussed in [20]. To compare the results from two laboratories, each laboratory received 25 samples of canola oil. Below are the fat content measurements (in %).

laboratory 1								
39.8	39.8	39.8	39.2	39.8	39.6	40.1	40.1	39.5
39.8	39.8	39.3	40.0	39.8	39.5	40.5	39.6	39.9
39.7	40.3	40.1	40.1	39.7	40.0	40.2		

laboratory 2								
40.0	39.9	39.7	39.5	39.6	39.6	39.7	39.8	40.1
39.4	39.0	39.5	40.3	39.2	40.0	39.2	39.7	39.7
39.7	39.5	39.8	40.0	39.4	39.5	39.5		

(a) Using a statistical software, verify the assumption that the two populations are normally distributed, with equal variances.
(b) Test the hypothesis $H_0 : \mu_1 = \mu_2$ versus $H_1 : \mu_1 \neq \mu_2$, where μ_1 is the average fat content from laboratory 1, and μ_2 is the average fat content from laboratory 2. State your conclusion. Use the level $\alpha = 0.05$.
(c) A difference in the means (in absolute value) is considered to be important, only if it is larger than 0.5. Construct a 95% confidence interval for $\mu_1 - \mu_2$. Is the difference between the means important?
Hint: For (b) and (c), you may approximate the $T(48)$ distribution with the standard normal distribution, or use a statistical software to find the exact probabilities associated with the $T(48)$ distribution.

Problem 16.20. Refer to Example 14.3. Let p_1 and p_2 be the proportions of cervical cancer cases in the vaccinated population, respectively the general population. Use a test of hypothesis for $H_0 : p_1 = p_2$ against $H_1 : p_1 < p_2$ to see if there is enough evidence that the vaccine is efficient in reducing the incidence of cervical cancer.

Problem 16.21. A study examines the weight loss of bears during hibernation. The study involves 18 bears of varying weights. For each bear, its weight (in kg) is measured during the month of November, and during the following month of March. The data are in the table below.

Bear	Fall Weight	Spring Weight	Bear	Fall Weight	Spring Weight
1	432.5	417.1	10	307.9	294.5
2	240.8	218.5	11	436.5	414.7
3	111.2	101.1	12	334.8	325.9
4	330.8	299.1	13	538.4	522.1
5	221.7	201.2	14	181.3	158.1
6	491.3	471.8	15	523.5	514.2
7	276.9	262.4	16	496.5	461.2
8	328.9	293.5	17	577.9	574.8
9	313.7	280.2	18	341.4	308.0

Is there any evidence that a bear will lose weight during hibernation? Justify your answer using a 95% confidence interval and a test of hypothesis. (Verify first that weight losses satisfy the normality assumption.)

Problem 16.22. The objective of the study [33] was to measure the association between a risk assessment for heart disease and the total coronary atherosclerotic plaque burden. The table below gives the cross-classification of the 1,653 subjects according to their risk category and their measure of coronary atherosclerosis severity (in terms of a segment plaque score).

Segment plaque score	Risk Category: Low	Intermediate	Moderately High	High
Zero	427	106	37	32
Mild	292	128	102	82
Moderate	108	50	85	58
Heavy	33	9	39	65

Is there an association between the segment plaque score and the risk category? Use the significance level $\alpha = 0.05$.

Problem 16.23. "Ottawa water usage spiked after Crosby scored golden goal, data show" is the title of an article that appeared in the Ottawa Citizen on March 17, 2010, written by Glen McGregor. Officials in many Canadian cities (including Ottawa, Edmonton and Vancouver) observed a spike in the water usage immediately after Sidney Crosby's winning goal that gave gold to Canada against the United States men's national hockey team at the Vancouver winter olympics in 2010. Canada is fortunate, since it has only 0.5% of the world's population, but its landmass contains approximately 7% of the world's renewable water supply (source: www.ec.gc.ca/eau-water).

Below are data of the water consumption (in million of litres) for a particular city in 50 randomly selected days.

281	282	287	288	289	289	291	291
291	291	292	293	293	293	293	294
294	294	294	295	297	297	297	297
297	298	299	301	301	301	302	303
303	304	304	305	306	307	307	307
308	309	310	310	311	312	312	314
315	322						

We summarize the data with the following two sums:

$$\sum_{i=1}^{50} x_i = 14,971 \quad \text{and} \quad \sum_{i=1}^{50} x_i^2 = 4,486,567.$$

(a) Using the above summary statistics compute the sample mean and the sample standard deviation.
(b) Find the median, and the two quartiles.
(c) Calculate the IQR. Are there any outliers?
(d) Produce a histogram of the data and describe the shape of the distribution.
(e) Construct a QQ-plot (or a normal probability plot). Does it appear reasonable to model the daily consumption of water with a normal distribution?

Did you know that? *The island of South Georgia in the south Atlantic Ocean is a sanctuary of wild life and an oasis in the stormy oceans surrounding Antarctica. The island is home to many species of birds, seals, penguins and reindeer, and during the breeding season, it hosts the densest population of marine animals on Earth. The island is a British overseas territory which was explored for the first time in 1775 by Captain James Cook, who brought back to England the news of an island full of seals. In the decades that followed, most species of seals were hunted to the verge of extinction. In the 20th century, the island became a whaling base, which contributed to the decay of the whale population in the waters nearby. In the recent years, as hunting became more tightly regulated, the seal and whale populations are making an incredible come back. The landscape of the island is stunningly beautiful, with snow covered peaks, and green bays. Half of the island is covered by permanent snow and ice, and the rest is covered by tundra vegetation. One can read more about this island in* [12].

Chapter 17

Tables

Table 17.1 Binomial coefficients $\binom{n}{k}$

	k					
n	0	1	2	3	4	5
1	1	1				
2	1	2	1			
3	1	3	3	1		
4	1	4	6	4	1	
5	1	5	10	10	5	1
6	1	6	15	20	15	6
7	1	7	21	35	35	21
8	1	8	28	56	70	56
9	1	9	36	84	126	126
10	1	10	45	120	210	252
11	1	11	55	165	330	462
12	1	12	66	220	495	792
13	1	13	78	286	715	1,287
14	1	14	91	364	1,001	2,002
15	1	15	105	455	1,365	3,003
16	1	16	120	560	1,820	4,368
17	1	17	136	680	2,380	6,188
18	1	18	153	816	3,060	8,568
19	1	19	171	969	3,876	11,628
20	1	20	190	1,140	4,845	15,504

	k				
n	6	7	8	9	10
6	1				
7	7	1			
8	28	8	1		
9	84	36	9	1	
10	210	120	45	10	1
11	462	330	165	55	11
12	924	792	495	220	66
13	1,716	1,716	1,287	715	286
14	3,003	3,432	3,003	2,002	1,001
15	5,005	6,435	6,435	5,005	3,003
16	8,008	11,440	12,870	11,440	8,008
17	12,376	19,448	24,310	24,310	19,448
18	18,564	31,824	43,758	48,620	43,758
19	27,132	50,388	75,582	92,378	92,378
20	38,760	77,520	125,970	167,960	184,756

Table 17.2 Cumulative probabilities for the standard normal: $\Phi(z) = P(Z \leq z)$

0.09	0.08	0.07	0.06	0.05	0.04	0.03	0.02	0.01	0.00	z
.0001	.0001	.0001	.0001	.0001	.0001	.0001	.0001	.0001	.0001	−3.8
.0001	.0001	.0001	.0001	.0001	.0001	.0001	.0001	.0001	.0001	−3.7
.0001	.0001	.0001	.0001	.0001	.0001	.0001	.0001	.0002	.0002	−3.6
.0002	.0002	.0002	.0002	.0002	.0002	.0002	.0002	.0002	.0002	−3.5
.0002	.0003	.0003	.0003	.0003	.0003	.0003	.0003	.0003	.0003	−3.4
.0003	.0004	.0004	.0004	.0004	.0004	.0004	.0005	.0005	.0005	−3.3
.0005	.0005	.0005	.0006	.0006	.0006	.0006	.0006	.0007	.0007	−3.2
.0007	.0007	.0008	.0008	.0008	.0008	.0009	.0009	.0009	.0010	−3.1
.0010	.0010	.0011	.0011	.0011	.0012	.0012	.0013	.0013	.0013	−3.0
.0014	.0014	.0015	.0015	.0016	.0016	.0017	.0018	.0018	.0019	−2.9
.0019	.0020	.0021	.0021	.0022	.0023	.0023	.0024	.0025	.0026	−2.8
.0026	.0027	.0028	.0029	.0030	.0031	.0032	.0033	.0034	.0035	−2.7
.0036	.0037	.0038	.0039	.0040	.0041	.0043	.0044	.0045	.0047	−2.6
.0048	.0049	.0051	.0052	.0054	.0055	.0057	.0059	.0060	.0062	−2.5
.0064	.0066	.0068	.0069	.0071	.0073	.0075	.0078	.0080	.0082	−2.4
.0084	.0087	.0089	.0091	.0094	.0096	.0099	.0102	.0104	.0107	−2.3
.0110	.0113	.0116	.0119	.0122	.0125	.0129	.0132	.0136	.0139	−2.2
.0143	.0146	.0150	.0154	.0158	.0162	.0166	.0170	.0174	.0179	−2.1
.0183	.0188	.0192	.0197	.0202	.0207	.0212	.0217	.0222	.0228	−2.0
.0233	.0239	.0244	.0250	.0256	.0262	.0268	.0274	.0281	.0287	−1.9
.0294	.0301	.0307	.0314	.0322	.0329	.0336	.0344	.0351	.0359	−1.8
.0367	.0375	.0384	.0392	.0401	.0409	.0418	.0427	.0436	.0446	−1.7
.0455	.0465	.0475	.0485	.0495	.0505	.0516	.0526	.0537	.0548	−1.6
.0559	.0571	.0582	.0594	.0606	.0618	.0630	.0643	.0655	.0668	−1.5
.0681	.0694	.0708	.0721	.0735	.0749	.0764	.0778	.0793	.0808	−1.4
.0823	.0838	.0853	.0869	.0885	.0901	.0918	.0934	.0951	.0968	−1.3
.0985	.1003	.1020	.1038	.1056	.1075	.1093	.1112	.1131	.1151	−1.2
.1170	.1190	.1210	.1230	.1251	.1271	.1292	.1314	.1335	.1357	−1.1
.1379	.1401	.1423	.1446	.1469	.1492	.1515	.1539	.1562	.1587	−1.0
.1611	.1635	.1660	.1685	.1711	.1736	.1762	.1788	.1814	.1841	−0.9
.1867	.1894	.1922	.1949	.1977	.2005	.2033	.2061	.2090	.2119	−0.8
.2148	.2177	.2206	.2236	.2266	.2296	.2327	.2358	.2389	.242	−0.7
.2451	.2483	.2514	.2546	.2578	.2611	.2643	.2676	.2709	.2743	−0.6
.2776	.2810	.2843	.2877	.2912	.2946	.2981	.3015	.3050	.3085	−0.5
.3121	.3156	.3192	.3228	.3264	.3300	.3336	.3372	.3409	.3446	−0.4
.3483	.3520	.3557	.3594	.3632	.3669	.3707	.3745	.3783	.3821	−0.3
.3859	.3897	.3936	.3974	.4013	.4052	.4090	.4129	.4168	.4207	−0.2
.4247	.4286	.4325	.4364	.4404	.4443	.4483	.4522	.4562	.4602	−0.1
.4641	.4681	.4721	.4761	.4801	.4840	.4880	.4920	.4960	.5000	−0.0

Table 17.3 Cumulative probabilities for the standard normal: $\Phi(z) = P(Z \leq z)$

z	0.00	0.01	0.02	0.03	0.04	0.05	0.06	0.07	0.08	0.09
0.0	.5000	.5040	.5080	.5120	.5160	.5199	.5239	.5279	.5319	.5359
0.1	.5398	.5438	.5478	.5517	.5557	.5596	.5636	.5675	.5714	.5753
0.2	.5793	.5832	.5871	.5910	.5948	.5987	.6026	.6064	.6103	.6141
0.3	.6179	.6217	.6255	.6293	.6331	.6368	.6406	.6443	.6480	.6517
0.4	.6554	.6591	.6628	.6664	.6700	.6736	.6772	.6808	.6844	.6879
0.5	.6915	.6950	.6985	.7019	.7054	.7088	.7123	.7157	.7190	.7224
0.6	.7257	.7291	.7324	.7357	.7389	.7422	.7454	.7486	.7517	.7549
0.7	.7580	.7611	.7642	.7673	.7704	.7734	.7764	.7794	.7823	.7852
0.8	.7881	.7910	.7939	.7967	.7995	.8023	.8051	.8078	.8106	.8133
0.9	.8159	.8186	.8212	.8238	.8264	.8289	.8315	.8340	.8365	.8389
1.0	.8413	.8438	.8461	.8485	.8508	.8531	.8554	.8577	.8599	.8621
1.1	.8643	.8665	.8686	.8708	.8729	.8749	.8770	.8790	.8810	.8830
1.2	.8849	.8869	.8888	.8907	.8925	.8944	.8962	.8980	.8997	.9015
1.3	.9032	.9049	.9066	.9082	.9099	.9115	.9131	.9147	.9162	.9177
1.4	.9192	.9207	.9222	.9236	.9251	.9265	.9279	.9292	.9306	.9319
1.5	.9332	.9345	.9357	.9370	.9382	.9394	.9406	.9418	.9429	.9441
1.6	.9452	.9463	.9474	.9484	.9495	.9505	.9515	.9525	.9535	.9545
1.7	.9554	.9564	.9573	.9582	.9591	.9599	.9608	.9616	.9625	.9633
1.8	.9641	.9649	.9656	.9664	.9671	.9678	.9686	.9693	.9699	.9706
1.9	.9713	.9719	.9726	.9732	.9738	.9744	.9750	.9756	.9761	.9767
2.0	.9772	.9778	.9783	.9788	.9793	.9798	.9803	.9808	.9812	.9817
2.1	.9821	.9826	.9830	.9834	.9838	.9842	.9846	.9850	.9854	.9857
2.2	.9861	.9864	.9868	.9871	.9875	.9878	.9881	.9884	.9887	.9890
2.3	.9893	.9896	.9898	.9901	.9904	.9906	.9909	.9911	.9913	.9916
2.4	.9918	.9920	.9922	.9925	.9927	.9929	.9931	.9932	.9934	.9936
2.5	.9938	.9940	.9941	.9943	.9945	.9946	.9948	.9949	.9951	.9952
2.6	.9953	.9955	.9956	.9957	.9959	.9960	.9961	.9962	.9963	.9964
2.7	.9965	.9966	.9967	.9968	.9969	.9970	.9971	.9972	.9973	.9974
2.8	.9974	.9975	.9976	.9977	.9977	.9978	.9979	.9979	.9980	.9981
2.9	.9981	.9982	.9982	.9983	.9984	.9984	.9985	.9985	.9986	.9986
3.0	.9987	.9987	.9987	.9988	.9988	.9989	.9989	.9989	.9990	.9990
3.1	.9990	.9991	.9991	.9991	.9992	.9992	.9992	.9992	.9993	.9993
3.2	.9993	.9993	.9994	.9994	.9994	.9994	.9994	.9995	.9995	.9995
3.3	.9995	.9995	.9995	.9996	.9996	.9996	.9996	.9996	.9996	.9997
3.4	.9997	.9997	.9997	.9997	.9997	.9997	.9997	.9997	.9997	.9998
3.5	.9998	.9998	.9998	.9998	.9998	.9998	.9998	.9998	.9998	.9998
3.6	.9998	.9998	.9999	.9999	.9999	.9999	.9999	.9999	.9999	.9999
3.7	.9999	.9999	.9999	.9999	.9999	.9999	.9999	.9999	.9999	.9999
3.8	.9999	.9999	.9999	.9999	.9999	.9999	.9999	.9999	.9999	.9999

Table 17.4 T distribution with ν degrees of freedom

$F_T(t) = P(T \leq t)$

	.6	.75	.9	.95	.975	.99	.995
ν	$t_{.40,\nu}$	$t_{.25,\nu}$	$t_{.10,\nu}$	$t_{.05,\nu}$	$t_{.025,\nu}$	$t_{.01,\nu}$	$t_{.005,\nu}$
1	0.325	1.000	3.078	6.314	12.706	31.821	63.657
2	0.289	0.816	1.886	2.920	4.303	6.965	9.925
3	0.277	0.765	1.638	2.353	3.182	4.541	5.841
4	0.271	0.741	1.533	2.132	2.776	3.747	4.604
5	0.267	0.727	1.476	2.015	2.571	3.365	4.032
6	0.265	0.718	1.440	1.943	2.447	3.143	3.707
7	0.263	0.711	1.415	1.895	2.365	2.998	3.499
8	0.262	0.706	1.397	1.860	2.306	2.896	3.355
9	0.261	0.703	1.383	1.833	2.262	2.821	3.250
10	0.260	0.700	1.372	1.812	2.228	2.764	3.169
11	0.260	0.697	1.363	1.796	2.201	2.718	3.106
12	0.259	0.695	1.356	1.782	2.179	2.681	3.055
13	0.259	0.694	1.350	1.771	2.160	2.650	3.012
14	0.258	0.692	1.345	1.761	2.145	2.624	2.997
15	0.258	0.691	1.341	1.753	2.131	2.602	2.947
16	0.258	0.690	1.337	1.746	2.120	2.583	2.921
17	0.257	0.689	1.333	1.740	2.110	2.567	2.898
18	0.257	0.688	1.330	1.734	2.101	2.552	2.878
19	0.257	0.688	1.328	1.729	2.093	2.539	2.861
20	0.257	0.687	1.325	1.725	2.086	2.528	2.845
21	0.257	0.686	1.323	1.721	2.080	2.518	2.831
22	0.256	0.686	1.321	1.717	2.074	2.508	2.819
23	0.256	0.685	1.319	1.714	2.069	2.500	2.807
24	0.256	0.685	1.318	1.711	2.064	2.492	2.797
25	0.256	0.684	1.316	1.708	2.060	2.485	2.787
26	0.256	0.684	1.315	1.706	2.056	2.479	2.779
27	0.256	0.684	1.314	1.703	2.052	2.473	2.771
28	0.256	0.683	1.313	1.701	2.048	2.467	2.763
29	0.256	0.683	1.311	1.699	2.045	2.464	2.756
30	0.256	0.683	1.310	1.697	2.042	2.457	2.750
∞	0.253	0.674	1.282	1.645	1.96	2.326	2.576

Note: $z_\alpha = t_{\alpha,\infty}$

Table 17.5 χ^2 distribution with ν degrees of freedom

$F_{\chi^2}(x) = P(\chi^2 \leq x)$

	0.5	0.75	0.9	0.95	0.975	0.99	0.995
ν	$\chi^2_{.50,\nu}$	$\chi^2_{.25,\nu}$	$\chi^2_{.10,\nu}$	$\chi^2_{.05,\nu}$	$\chi^2_{.025,\nu}$	$\chi^2_{.01,\nu}$	$\chi^2_{.005,\nu}$
1	0.455	1.323	2.706	3.841	5.024	6.635	7.879
2	1.386	2.773	4.605	5.991	7.378	9.21	10.60
3	2.366	4.108	6.251	7.815	9.348	11.345	12.84
4	3.357	5.385	7.779	9.488	11.14	13.277	14.86
5	4.351	6.626	9.236	11.07	12.83	15.086	16.75
6	5.348	7.841	10.65	12.59	14.45	16.81	18.55
7	6.346	9.037	12.02	14.07	16.01	18.48	20.28
8	7.344	10.22	13.36	15.51	17.54	20.09	21.96
9	8.343	11.39	14.68	16.92	19.02	21.67	23.59
10	9.342	12.55	15.99	18.31	20.48	23.21	25.19
11	10.34	13.70	17.28	19.68	21.92	24.73	26.76
12	11.34	14.85	18.55	21.03	23.34	26.22	28.30
13	12.34	15.98	19.81	22.36	24.74	27.69	29.82
14	13.34	17.12	21.06	23.69	26.12	29.14	31.32
15	14.34	18.25	22.31	25.00	27.49	30.58	32.80
16	15.34	19.37	23.54	26.30	28.85	32.00	34.27
17	16.34	20.49	24.77	27.59	30.19	33.41	35.72
18	17.34	21.61	25.99	28.87	31.53	34.81	37.16
19	18.34	22.72	27.20	30.14	32.85	36.19	38.58
20	19.34	23.83	28.41	31.41	34.17	37.57	40.00
21	20.34	24.94	29.62	32.67	35.48	38.93	41.40
22	21.34	26.04	30.81	33.92	36.78	40.29	42.80
23	22.34	27.14	32.01	35.17	38.08	41.64	44.18
24	23.34	28.24	33.20	36.42	39.36	42.98	45.56
25	24.34	29.34	34.38	37.65	40.65	44.31	46.93
26	25.34	30.44	35.56	38.89	41.92	45.64	48.29
27	26.34	31.53	36.74	40.11	43.20	46.96	49.65
28	27.34	32.62	37.92	41.34	44.46	48.28	50.99
29	28.34	33.71	39.09	42.56	45.72	49.59	52.34
30	29.34	34.80	40.26	43.77	46.98	50.89	53.67
31	30.34	35.89	41.42	44.99	48.23	52.19	55.00
32	31.34	36.97	42.59	46.19	49.48	53.49	56.33
33	32.34	38.06	43.75	47.40	50.73	54.78	57.65
34	33.34	39.14	44.90	48.60	51.97	56.06	58.96
35	34.34	40.22	46.06	49.80	53.20	57.34	60.28

Bibliography

[1] Albert, D. M. and Bowyer, R. T. (1991). Factors related to grizzly bear: Human Interactions in Denali National Park, *Wildlife Society Bulletin* **19**, pp. 339–349.

[2] Allen, G. E. (1978). *Thomas Hunt Morgan : the man and his science* (Princeton University Press).

[3] Ancker, J. S. (2006). The Language of conditional probability, *Journal of Statistics Education. [Online]* **14**, http://www.amstat.org/publications/jse/v14n2/ancker.html.

[4] Andersson, M. L., Roos, E. M., Petersson, I. F., Heinegard, D. and Saxne, T. (2006). Serum levels of Cartilage Oligomeric Matrix Protein (COMP) increase temporarily after physical exercise in patients with knee osteoarthritis, *BMC Musculoskelet Disord* **7**, pp. 1471–1474.

[5] Ary, D. V., Lichtenstein, E., Severson, H., Weissman, W., and Seeley, J. R. (1989). An in-depth analysis of male adolescent smokeless tobacco users: interviews with users and their fathers, *Journal of Behavioral Medicine* **12**, pp. 449–467.

[6] Asimov, I. (1964). *Adding a Dimension. Seventeen Essays on the History of Science* (Doubleday & Company).

[7] Ayanlade, A., Babatimehin, O., Olawole, M.O. and Orimogunje, O. O. I. (2010). Geospatial quality data acquisition problems in sub-Saharan Africa, *Journal of Sustainable Development in Africa* **12**, pp. 146–152.

[8] Batten, M. (1968). *Discovery by Chance. Science and the Unexpected* (Funk and Wagnalls).

[9] Bawa, K. S., Kang, H. and Grayum, M. H. (2003). Relationships among time, frequency, and duration of flowering in tropical rain forest trees, *American Journal of Botany* **90**, pp. 877–887.

[10] Bednarek, R. and Davidson, C. S. (1967). Influence of spraying with carbaryl on nesting success in a sample of bird-boxes on cape cod in 1965, *Bird Banding* **38**, pp. 66–72.

[11] Bozeman, W. P. (2009). Additional information on taser safety, *Annals of Emergency Medicine* **54**, pp. 758–759.

[12] Brower, K. (2009). Resurrection island, *National Geographic* **12**, pp. 56–77.

[13] Chobanian A. V., Bakris G. L., Black H. R., et al. (2003). Seventh report of the joint national committee on prevention, detection, evaluation, and treatment of high blood pressure, *Hypertension* **42**, pp. 1206–1252.

[14] Claggett, M., Shrock, J. and Noll, K. E. (1981). Carbon monoxide near an urban intersection, *Atmospheric Environment* **15**, pp. 1633–1642.

[15] Carrasco, J. L., Daz-Marsà M., Hollander, E., César, J. and Saiz-Ruiz, J. (2000). Decreased platelet monoamine oxidase activity in female bulimia nervosa, *European Neuropsychopharmacology* **10**, pp. 113–117.

[16] Corbett, E. L., Watt, C. J. and Walker, N. (2003). The growing burden of tuberculosis: global trends and interactions with the HIV epidemics, *Archives of Internal Medicine* **163**, pp. 1009–1021.

[17] Davis, S., Mirick, D.K. and Stevens, R. G. (2001). Night shift work, light at night, and risk of breast cancer, *Journal of National Cancer Institute* **93**, pp. 1557–1562.

[18] Dooner, H. K., Robbins, T. P., and Jorgensen, R. A. (1991). Genetic and developmental control of anthocyanin biosynthesis, *Annual Review of Genetics* **25**, pp. 173-199.

[19] Dudewicz, E. J., Yan, M., Mai, E. and Su, H. (2007). Exact solutions to the Behrens-Fisher problem: asymptocially optimal and finite sample efficient choice among, *Journal of Statistical Planning and Inference* **137**, pp. 1584–1605.

[20] Eller, F. J. and King, J. W. (1996). Determination of fat content in foods by analytical SFE, *Seminars in Food Analysis* **1**, pp. 145–162.

[21] Fearon, K. C. H., Plumb, J. A., Burns, H. J. G. and Calman, K. C. (1987). Reduction of the growth rate of the Walker 256 tumor in rats by Rhodamine 6G together with hypoglycemia, *Cancer Research* **47**, pp. 3684–3687.

[22] Gardiner, B. G. (1984). Sturgeons as living fossils. In: *Living Fossils* (Eldridge, N. and Stanley, S. M. eds.), pp. 148–152.

[23] Garfinkel, A. et. al. (1999). Prognostic value of dobutamine dtress echocardiography in predicting cardiac events in patients with known or suspected coronary artery disease, *Journal of the American College of Cardiology* **33**, pp. 708–716.

[24] Garland, S.M., Hernandez-Avila, M., Wheeler, C. M. et al. (2007). Quadrivalent vaccine agians human Papillomavirus to prevent anogenital diseases, *New England Journal of Medicine* **356**, pp. 1928–1943.

[25] Gavish, B., Ben-Dov I. Z., Bursztyn M. (2008). Linear relationship between systolic and diastolic blood pressure monitored over 24 h: assessment and correlates, *Journal of Hypertension* **26**, pp. 199–209.

[26] Goodall, J. (1988). *My Life with Wild Chimpanzees* (Pocket Book).

[27] Guttman, B., Griffiths, A., Suzuki, D., and Cullis, T. (2002). *Genetics: A Beginner's Guide* (Oneworld Publications).

[28] Ha, A., Bae, S. and Urrutia-Rojas, X., Singh, K. P. (2005). Eating and physical activity practices in risk of overweight and overweight children, *Nutrition Research* **25**, pp. 905–915.

[29] Hagberg, J. M., Ehsani, A. A. and Holloszy, J. O. (1983). Effect of 12 months of intense exercise training on stroke volume in patients with coronary artery

disease, *Circulation* **67**, pp. 1194–1199.
[30] Hilderbrand, G. V., Hanley, T. A., Robbins, C. T. and Schwartz, C. C. (1999). Role of brown bears (Ursus arctos) in the flow of marine nitrogen into a terrestrial ecosystem, *Oecologia* **121**, pp. 546–550.
[31] Holland, J. (2010). Counting cranes, *National Geographic* **6**, pp. 68–79.
[32] Ingram, V. M. (1957). Gene mutations in human haemoglobin: the chemical difference between normal and sickle cell haemoglobin, *Nature* **180**, pp. 326–328.
[33] Johnson, K. M., Dowe, D. A. and Brink, J. A. (2009). Traditional clinical risk assessment tools do not accurately predict coronary atherosclerotic plaque burden: A CT angiography study, *American Journal of Roentgenology* **192**, pp. 235–243.
[34] Jurado, E. and Westoby, M. (1992). Germination biology of selected central Australian plants, *Australian Journal of Ecology* **17**, pp. 341–348.
[35] Kettlewell, H.B.D. (1959). Darwin's Missing Evidence, *Scientific American* **200**, pp. 48–53.
[36] Knoke, T. (2003). Predicting red heartwood formation in beech trees (Fagus sylvatica L.), *Ecological Modelling* **169**, pp. 295–312.
[37] Lally, S.P. (1999). Henry Cavendish and the density of the earth, *The Physics Teacher* **37**, pp. 34–37.
[38] Landauer, W. and Dunn, L. G. (1930). The "frizzle" character of fowls, *Journal of Heredity* **21**, pp. 291–305.
[39] Logson, S., Clay, D., Moore, D. and Tsegaye, T. (2008). *Soil Science: Step-by-Step Field Analysis* (Soil Science Society of America).
[40] Miko, I. (2008). Epistasis: gene interaction and phenotype effects, *Nature Education* **1**.
[41] Niculescu, T., Dumitru, R., Botha, V., Alexandrescu, R., and Manolescu, N. (1983). Relationship between the lead concentration in hair and occupational exposure, *British Journal of Industrial Medicine*, **40**, pp. 67–70.
[42] Nelson, J. L. ,Roeder, B. L. , Carmen, J. C. Roloff, F. and Pitt, W. G. (2002). Ultrasonically activated chemotherapeutic drug delivery in a rat model, *Cancer Research* **62**, pp. 7280–7283.
[43] Lange, P., Groth, S., Nyboe, G.J. et al. (1989). Effects of smoking and changes in smoking habits on the decline of FEV_1, *Eurupean Respiratory Journal* **2**, pp. 811–816.
[44] Lowe, A. J., Carlin, J. B., Bennett et al. (2010). Paracetamol use in early life and asthma: prospective birth cohort study, *British Medical Journal.* To appear.
[45] Paul, P. (2003). Medical opinion, *American Demographics* **6**.
[46] Pearl, R. (1914). The service and importance of statistics to biology, *Publications of the American Statistical Association* **14**, pp. 40–48.
[47] Poot, H., Ens, B. J., de Vries, H., Donners, M. A. H., Wernand, M. R., and Marquenie, J. M. (2008). Green light for nocturnally migrating birds, *Ecology and Society* **13**, pp. 47.
[48] Quammen, D. (2009). Darwin's first clues, *The National Geographic* **2**, pp. 34–55.

[49] Rothman, K. J., Greendland, S. and Lash, T. L. (2008). *Modern Epidemiology*, third edition (Lippincott Williams and Wilkins).

[50] Sakamoto, M., Hishioka, K. and Shimada, K (1979). Effect of malnutrition and nutritional rehabilitation on tuberculin reactivity and complement level in rats, *Immunology* **38**, pp. 413–420.

[51] Schartz, C. C., Miller, S. D. and Haroldson, M. A. (2003). Grizzly bear, in: *Wild Mammals of North America: Biology, Management, and Conservation*, G.A. Feldhamer, B.C. Thompson, and J.A. Chapman, eds., second edition (Johns Hopkins University Press) pp. 556–586.

[52] Stigler, S. M. (1977). Do robust estimators work with real data? *Annals of Statistics* **5**, pp. 1055–1098.

[53] Stirling, I. and Derocher, A. E. (2007). Melting under pressure: the real scoop on climate warming and polar bears, *The Wildlife Professional Spring* **43**, pp. 23–27.

[54] Sturtevant, A. H. (1913). The linear arrangement of six sex-linked factors in Drosophila, as shown by their mode of association, *Journal of Experimental Zoology* **14**, pp. 43-59.

[55] Tarburton, M. K. (1993). A comparison of the breeding biology of the Welcome Swallow in Australia and recently colonised New Zealand, *Emu* **93**, pp. 34-43.

[56] Teran, E., Hernandez, I., Nieto, B., Tavara, R., Ocampo, J. E. and Calle, A. (2009). Coenzyme Q10 supplementation during pregnancy reduces the risk of pre-eclampsia, *International Journal of Gynecology and Obstretics* **105**, pp. 43-45.

[57] Thomas, J. F. J. (1953). Industrial water resources of Canada, Water Survey Report No. 1. Scope, procedure, and interpretation of survey studies (Queen's Printer).

[58] Villeneuve, P. J. and Mao, Y. (1994). Lifetime probability of developing lung cancer, by smoking status, in Canada, *Canadian Journal of Public Health* **85**, pp. 385–388.

[59] Vincent, W. F., Gibson, J. A. E., Jeffries, M. O. (2001). Ice-shelf collapse, climate change, and habitat loss in the Canadian high Arctic, *Polar Record* **37**, pp. 133–142.

[60] Wann, E. V. and Hills, W. A. (1973). The genetics of boron and iron transport in the tomato, *Journal of Heredity* **64**, pp. 370–371.

[61] Welch, B. L. (1938). The significance of the difference between two means when the population variances are unequal, *Biometrika* **29**, pp. 350–361.

[62] Willis, C. M., Reiche, L. and Wilkinson, J. D. (1998). Immunocytochemical demonstration of reduced Cu,Zn-superoxide dismutase levels following topical application of dithranol and sodium lauryl sulphate: an indication of the role of oxidative stress in acute irritant contact dermatitis, *European Journal of Dermatology* **8**, pp. 8–12.

[63] Wojcinski, Z. W., Barker, I. K., Hunter, D. B., and Lumsden, H. (1987). An outbreak of schistosomiasis in Atlantic brant geese (Branta Bernicla Hrota), *Wildlife Disease Association* **23**, pp. 248–255.

T distribution with ν degrees of freedom

	$F_T(t) = P(T \leq t)$						
	.6	.75	.9	.95	.975	.99	.995
ν	$t_{.40,\nu}$	$t_{.25,\nu}$	$t_{.10,\nu}$	$t_{.05,\nu}$	$t_{.025,\nu}$	$t_{.01,\nu}$	$t_{.005,\nu}$
1	0.325	1.000	3.078	6.314	12.706	31.821	63.657
2	0.289	0.816	1.886	2.920	4.303	6.965	9.925
3	0.277	0.765	1.638	2.353	3.182	4.541	5.841
4	0.271	0.741	1.533	2.132	2.776	3.747	4.604
5	0.267	0.727	1.476	2.015	2.571	3.365	4.032
6	0.265	0.718	1.440	1.943	2.447	3.143	3.707
7	0.263	0.711	1.415	1.895	2.365	2.998	3.499
8	0.262	0.706	1.397	1.860	2.306	2.896	3.355
9	0.261	0.703	1.383	1.833	2.262	2.821	3.250
10	0.260	0.700	1.372	1.812	2.228	2.764	3.169
11	0.260	0.697	1.363	1.796	2.201	2.718	3.106
12	0.259	0.695	1.356	1.782	2.179	2.681	3.055
13	0.259	0.694	1.350	1.771	2.160	2.650	3.012
14	0.258	0.692	1.345	1.761	2.145	2.624	2.997
15	0.258	0.691	1.341	1.753	2.131	2.602	2.947
16	0.258	0.690	1.337	1.746	2.120	2.583	2.921
17	0.257	0.689	1.333	1.740	2.110	2.567	2.898
18	0.257	0.688	1.330	1.734	2.101	2.552	2.878
19	0.257	0.688	1.328	1.729	2.093	2.539	2.861
20	0.257	0.687	1.325	1.725	2.086	2.528	2.845
21	0.257	0.686	1.323	1.721	2.080	2.518	2.831
22	0.256	0.686	1.321	1.717	2.074	2.508	2.819
23	0.256	0.685	1.319	1.714	2.069	2.500	2.807
24	0.256	0.685	1.318	1.711	2.064	2.492	2.797
25	0.256	0.684	1.316	1.708	2.060	2.485	2.787
26	0.256	0.684	1.315	1.706	2.056	2.479	2.779
27	0.256	0.684	1.314	1.703	2.052	2.473	2.771
28	0.256	0.683	1.313	1.701	2.048	2.467	2.763
29	0.256	0.683	1.311	1.699	2.045	2.464	2.756
30	0.256	0.683	1.310	1.697	2.042	2.457	2.750
∞	0.253	0.674	1.282	1.645	1.96	2.326	2.576

Note: $z_\alpha = t_{\alpha,\infty}$